M383

14.95

Rotherham Health Care Library

B000976

D1103015

36322
(3)

Tel. 824525.
RSL
laminate

4 FEB 1993			
1995			
2 5 JUN 1996			
15 MAY 1997			
7/6 3/7			
5 NOV 1997			
21 APR 1998			
1 4 APR 2005			
1 9 MAY 2015			

WITHDRAWN FROM
ROTHERHAM NFT LIBRARY
ROTHERHAM HEALTH CARE
STAFF LIBRARY AND
& KNOWLEDGE SERVICE
INFORMATION SERVICE

You should aspire to the same standard of care you would expect for yourself or your family
—EXCELLENCE

Beyond First Aid

A skills-based guide to ambulance practice

921771

Peter Hewett
Co-ordinator, Associate Diploma Health Science (Ambulance Officer)
Ambulance Officers' Training Centre, Victoria

UK Advisers
John Oakden
Assistant Director Training, London Ambulance Service

Don Parsons
Area Manager, London Ambulance Service

Foreword by
Jeff Wassertheil SB StJ, MB BS, FACEM
Director, Department of Emergency Medicine, Epworth Hospital, Melbourne

CHURCHILL LIVINGSTONE
MELBOURNE EDINBURGH LONDON MADRID NEW YORK AND TOKYO

CHURCHILL LIVINGSTONE
Medical Division of Longman Group UK Limited

Distributed in Australia by Longman Cheshire Pty Limited, Longman House, Kings Gardens, 95 Coventry Street, South Melbourne 3205, and by associated companies, branches and representatives throughout the world.

© Longman Group UK Limited 1992

All rights reserved. No part of this publication may be reproduced, stored in a retrieval system, or transmitted in any form or by any means, electronic, mechanical, photo-copying, recording or otherwise, without the prior permission of the publishers (Churchill Livingstone, Robert Stevenson House, 1-3 Baxter's Place, Leith Walk, Edinburgh EH1 3AF), or a licence permitting restricted copying in the United Kingdom issued by the Copyright Licensing Agency Ltd, 90 Tottenham Court Road, London, W1P 9HE.

First published 1992

ISBN 0-443-04579-8

National Library of Australia Cataloguing in Publication Data

Hewett, Peter (Peter R.).
    Beyond first aid: a skills-based guide to ambulance practice.

    Includes index.
    ISBN 0 443 04579 8.

    1. Emergency medicine. 2. Ambulance service. I. Title.

616.025

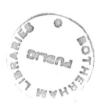

ROTHERHAM PUBLIC LIBRARIES

Produced by Longman Singapore Publishers (Pte) Ltd

Printed in Singapore

Foreword

I am honoured to have been asked to write the Foreword of this book. In doing so I am mindful of the significant changes that have taken place in pre-hospital patient management over the last two decades. During my undergraduate years I spent my vacation as a medical student ambulance officer. On reflection, that experience has certainly been an important influence on my own medical career.

When I was taught first aid, it was largely a theoretical subject which was supplemented by the demonstration of practical skills. Edict was the essence. One did not require much in the way of conceptual grasp of the principles behind the practice. It was often supported by handy tips and some unfounded, often inappropriate procedures. Ambulance personnel were little more qualified than a very good lay first aider. However, somewhat more training was needed for familiarisation with specialised equipment. Although the essentials were there, training was procedure orientated rather than holistic in approach and logically flowing.

The title *Beyond First Aid* suggests that traditional boundaries have been breached. Not only have they been breached from within the first aider environment, the horizon has been extended to, and within, the emergency facility with which ambulance intimately relates. Through all this, we have seen the evolution and maturation of ambulance officers and ambulance expertise. Adequate is not good enough. A sound understanding of the pathophysiological principles needs to be acquired and then applied to situations that confront ambulance personnel. Once this has been attained, the key to effective performance in the field is the mastery of skills as opposed to satisfactory performance. Mastery combined with repetition enhances performance. This in conjunction with skills maintenance strategies leads to proficiency.

It does not stop there. The essence of being a practitioner is the capacity to recognise patterns of presentation. Recognition cannot be taught. It is acquired by recurrent exposure to the various scenarios and situations requiring assessment and intervention. Training prepares the individual. 'Experience' is the end product of 'hands on' repeated again and again and again.

The complexity of skill development in the ambulance officer is further highlighted by the need to manage, at little or no notice, not only one, but several patients simultaneously. This also requires, through specific training and experience, the capacity to prioritise. The concept and practice is not new. Although the strategies were employed in the Gulf War in 1991, they date back to Napoleonic times, when triage was first implemented in the field for the multiple victim or mass casualty situation. Such decision making causes discomfort in lesser trained and experienced health care providers. Sometimes those who should be treated first on primary survey and vital signs criteria are least likely to survive and must be left, thus directing one's attention to victims who will survive. If they can be identified expediently, such victims may be taken to facilities that can intervene efficiently with relatively minimal delay.

In the early 1970s coronary care capability was brought to the patient in the home, public places, the workplace and in the street. This new perspective meant that the individual with acute myocardial infarction or cardiac arrest was being offered more than basic life support. Now, rapid response defibrillation is considered as part of the undergraduate training of ambulance personnel in many parts of the world. Advanced cardiac life support technology and skills have been expanded over the last decade resulting in the evolution of the paramedic.

Beyond First Aid does indeed take the new recruit by the hand through the essentials of first aid, and basic principles of emergency medicine; it mentors the student to achieving the knowledge and skills demanded by the training process. Proficiency it cannot teach. Proficiency also does not just happen. It requires motivation to gain as much exposure as possible to the varied situations the accomplished practitioner needs to master.

Jeff Wassertheil   June 1991

Preface

Emergency medicine is a relatively new medical specialty. It has developed from the critical care procedures used in anaesthesia and intensive care and to a significant extent, from the experiences of the Korean and Vietnam wars.

For many years, ambulance services have provided transport for the sick and injured, with a limited amount of on-site and in-transit care, based on the principles of first-aid. Today, the community expects a greater degree of sophistication and an ambulance system capable of rapid response and expert in pre-hospital care.

Since the early 1960s, ambulance services have evolved into a specialised branch of the health system, through formal training programs which go beyond the boundaries of first-aid, with access to sophisticated, portable technology. But regardless of this technological explosion, the basic principles of first-aid and emergency care, the 'hands on' skills, must still be maintained as the cornerstone to pre-hospital management.

There are many texts written on pre-hospital care, covering the principles and practice in both basic life support and advanced care. The bulk of this book is practically oriented, with the aim of providing a common sense, competency-based learning guide. Each chapter specifies tasks for the student to practise, and refers him or her on to the step-by-step descriptions of the relevant procedures and techniques at the back of the book. These skills guides can be readily adapted by individual ambulance services to their own equipment and methods of patient care.

Basic life support, the life essential skills and procedures, are considered first. Anatomy and physiology are included in outline only and I recommend that a more detailed text be used in conjunction with this book.

Advanced life support concepts and practices are developed in Chapter 9 as an extension to basic principles. Before attempting to master these new skills, it is vital to ensure your own basic skills are more than satisfactory. In addition to technical proficiency, it is important to remember as well that you are caring for a person who has the same feelings, wants and needs as you. They must be treated as a 'whole' being, both emotionally and physically.

Melbourne 1991   Peter Hewett

Acknowledgements

This text has been written as a result of many years of collecting and preparing student notes for training programmes in ambulance operations. Much of the material is based on notes prepared in collaboration with my colleagues at the Ambulance Officers Training Centre in Melbourne. Their support and kindness is greatly appreciated. I especially thank Dr Frank Archer, Ambulance Services Medical Officer, a colleague and valued friend with whom some of this material was written; Beata Csupor, Critical Care Nurse and mobile intensive care lecturer at AOTC, for assistance with information in the ALS area; David Dawson, psychologist and teaching colleague, for his valuable help with the behavioural material. I am most grateful for the assistance of Mr Peter Newbold, Executive Director, AOTC, for allowing me the freedom to write this text and have access to material, and to Dr Jeff Wassertheil, for patiently reading my drafts and critiquing the text.

To the ambulance officers who assisted me with the illustrations—Mark Bruere, Mark Chilton, Ian Clark, Graham Fitton, Brendan Holman, Debra Kelly, Mark MacCreedie, Robyn Oliphant and Phil White—my thanks. I am most grateful for the assistance of Mr John Oakden, Assistant Director Training, and Mr Don Parsons, Area Manager, of the London Ambulance Service.

I would also like to thank my publishers Churchill Livingstone for permission to reproduce diagrams from Kathleen J W Wilson's Ross & Wilson, Anatomy and Physiology in Health and Illness (seventh edition), and the Victorian Ambulance Services Association for permission to reproduce parts of its patient care record form.

To Judy Waters and John Macdonald of Churchill Livingstone, whose skills and experience in producing textbooks have been invaluable, I sincerely thank them for their patience, encouragement and support to make this text possible.

Finally, to Michelle, Melissa and Brad, my family, who have put up with much during the long period of writing and editing, my love and thanks for their support.

P.R.H.

Contents

Guide to using the text

The aim of the text is to assist you to develop competence in the skills of ambulance practice. Each chapter deals with a range of skills and presents supporting information to increase your understanding of the processes and responses of the body in crisis.

A learning guide is provided for each segment of the chapter to help you plan studies and activities. These include performing the relevant tasks, which are specified in each chapter. Knowledge checks assist you in checking your progress before continuing. Skills guides are provided for each task and can be located after page 237. A case history with questions is presented in each of the clinical chapters to help you to consolidate your learning. The answers to the knowledge checks and case histories can be found on page 299.

SECTION 1
Introduction to practice

CHAPTER 1
Before we start

Before exploring clinical problems and the application of technology, there are a few issues to consider. Preparation for working in the ambulance environment involves attention to both physical and emotional development as well as the knowledge and skills of clinical practice.

Personal fitness and health are important in reducing the risks of injury. Safe lifting and other occupational health and safety considerations are imperative. In a caring profession, we spend a large portion of our time dealing with the crises of other individuals, families and groups. We need to realise that we are not immune from the emotional turmoils of violence and death and may need to look for coping strategies and personal help.

Topics covered

Personal fitness and health
Safe lifting
Environmental hazards
Dealing with job demands
Driving an emergency vehicle
Medico-legal considerations

The modern concept of pre-hospital care had its origins in Europe in the latter half of the 18th century. The first teaching of expired air resuscitation to the lay public commenced in Amsterdam in 1767, followed by the formation of the Royal Humane Society in London in 1774.

Napoleon's Surgeon General, Dominic Jean Larrey, during his appointment to the Army of the Rhine in 1792, developed the concept of immediate care on the field of combat, with his idea of an ambulance—which he described as both a field hospital, and a conveyance for wounded soldiers. Transport was by wheeled stretcher and a horse-drawn light ambulance carriage, with seriously injured soldiers being given life-saving first aid where they fell.

In the late 1960s, almost 200 years after Larrey, pre-hospital care moved into the technological age. 'Paramedic' services and developments in pre-hospital 'advanced life support' emerged, using sophisticated portable technology and the principles of care from the hospital emergency department and intensive care. Despite the technological explosion and sophistication of today's ambulance services, the basic principles of first aid and Larrey's concept 'stabilise before transport' survive as the cornerstones of pre-hospital patient care.

The primary role of the ambulance officer is to provide emergency care in cases of accident and acute illness and health transport to a medical facility. This role requires the officer to lift and carry injured and sick people, operate a motor vehicle—at times, at higher speeds than normal traffic flow—and not infrequently cope with crisis situations, involving death and gross injury. Preparation for working in such an environment—which is sometimes hostile—must therefore require attention to both physical and emotional development, skills and knowledge of safe lifting methods, an understanding of the hazards encountered in the environment, and an ability to communicate and empathise with all people—not only the patient. However, despite what you might see on television, the greatest percentage of ambulance operational duty is non-emergency, routine health transport.

PERSONAL FITNESS AND HEALTH

Much has been written about physical fitness and life-style with regard to preventing heart disease and other degenerative disease processes. Technological changes have reduced the need for physical work in modern society and this can probably be linked with the higher incidence of back injury and other occupational problems in the community. Despite the advent of improved lifting devices and more efficient stretchers, which minimise the physical work required to convey a patient, there is still an important need for you to maintain a good level of physical fitness in order to be capable of performing tasks safely, thus reducing the risk of personal injury.

SAFE LIFTING

Aim
To develop an understanding of prevention of back injury and to develop skills in safe lifting

Learning plan
1. Read the text information
2. Practise the safe lifting skills using the skills guides to check your progress

Statistics demonstrate a high incidence of back injury in our society and ambulance officers are not excluded. The sedentary nature of the job, interspersed with short episodes of physical work, creates an occupational risk. Situations in which back strain occurs may not produce immediate recognisable problems, but progressive aggravation through frequent lifting ultimately leads to serious disability.

Back pain and injury are most commonly the result of

- Unaccustomed exercise, which places an unusual strain on muscles which are not properly conditioned
- Sudden and violent stretching of muscles
- Improper use of muscles, through poor lifting and handling methods.

The risks can be reduced significantly by maintaining a good level of fitness and being conscious of posture and movements on the job.

1

Guide to preventing back strain

1. Size up the job—get help if the load appears too heavy or awkward
2. Check your footing—don't take a chance on falling
3. Face the job—avoid twisting when lifting
4. Distribute weight evenly for good balance—spread feet about shoulder width apart, or alternatively one foot beside and the other behind the object
5. Squat, don't bend, to working level—bend your knees; keep your back straight, not vertical (there is a difference)
6. Lift with your legs, not your back—push up with the strong leg muscles
7. Carry the weight as close to your body as practicable
8. Don't twist your body—to change direction, shift your foot position
9. Work together when team lifting—work on a signal from a designated leader
10. Bend your knees to lower the load

Posture (or rather the lack of it) is a potential cause of back pain. Given that the role of the ambulance officer often requires long periods driving the vehicle, the maintenance of good posture is a simple but sound preventive practice. Make sure that your seat is adjusted to support the natural arch of the spine and does not permit slumping. Sitting well back into the seat will reduce the space between your spine and back support. A comfortable, well balanced sitting position is not only a good preventive measure against back pain, but also reduces fatigue and improves the duration of concentration.

LIFTING SKILLS

Manual techniques

Manual lifting procedures require the use of two rescuers. The most commonly used lifting procedure is a fore-and-aft lift (Fig. 1.1).

Indications

The sitting patient without upper limb or trunk injury. Can be used to move an unconscious patient if the rescuers can move the patient safely into a sitting position.

Precautions

Avoid placing yourself in a position where your body is twisted, e.g., through the doorway of a motor vehicle.

Attempting flat lifting in the pre-hospital care environment is risking personal injury, regardless of how many people are available to help and should not be used. Moving a patient from the roadside or the floor to a stretcher is more safely achieved by using a lifting device. If no device is available, a blanket is an ideal means of moving the patient. It can be easily positioned under the patient and provides a safe and comfortable means to grip and lift.

| **TASK** | Lift a patient using the fore-and-aft method | **240** |

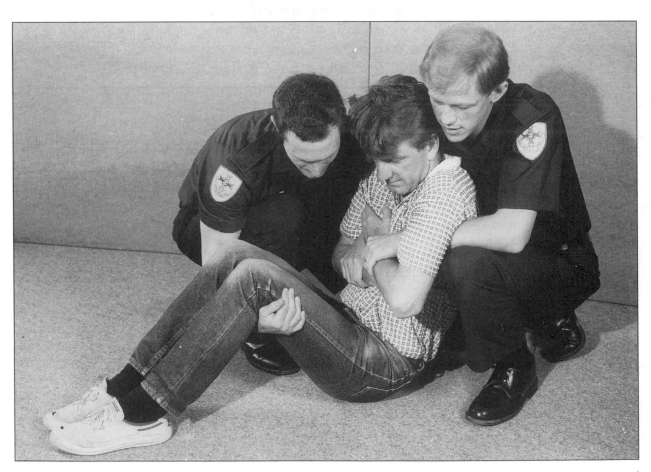

Fig. 1.1 Fore-and-aft lift. The two rescuers must be in balance and lift together slowly.

Lifting devices

There are several pieces of apparatus used in pre-hospital care. In some services, back boards are employed, while others utilise specially designed lifting frames, e.g., the Jordon Lifting Frame (Fig. 1.2).

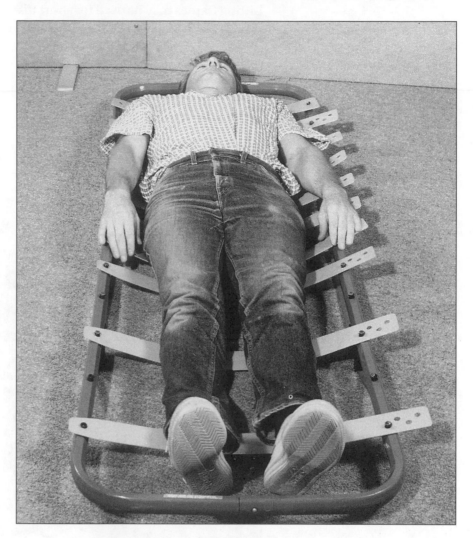

Fig. 1.2 The Jordon Lifting Frame is assembled around the patient. Take care that the gliders are fastened securely to the same side. Think about which side the stretcher will be placed in the ambulance.

Frames, with detachable glider supports, are versatile and can be used in most situations, especially where the surface on which the patient is located is uneven or loose.

There are also orthopaedic stretchers specifically designed to gently scoop under the patient using a scissor-type motion, e.g., the Scoop stretcher. The open centre of these stretchers allows X ray of the vertebral column without moving the patient.

Care should always be taken with any firm lifting device to minimise the pressure on soft tissues, especially where the patient remains on such a device for long periods.

Indications

Lifting from a flat position, where maintenance of the patient's position is necessary, e.g., spinal injury or multiple injury. Moving a patient in situations where manual methods place the rescuer at risk of personal injury.

Precautions

Ensure that the patient is secure before lifting. Make certain that it is possible to manoeuvre the patient safely to the stretcher before using the device.

Lifting frames may be used for short distance where the main stretcher cannot be used,. However, such devices are not designed for carrying. In the major incident setting, where emergency evacuation of patients from hazards is necessary, temporary restraint may be required to avoid the risk of further injury to the patient.

TASK	Lift a patient using a lifting frame	244

Chair lift

In some circumstances, it is not possible to position a stretcher near the patient and the access from the site is difficult, e.g., where awkward

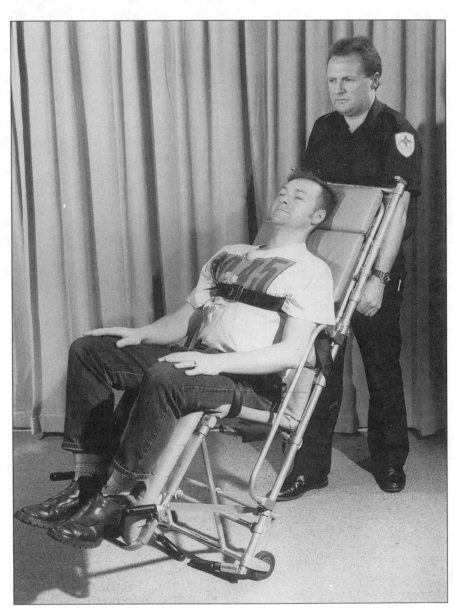

Fig. 1.3 When using the carry chair, always secure the patient .

corners or stairs have to be negotiated. Many stretchers in use today consist of a detachable stretcher and trolley.

Some of these stretchers are designed to fold into a chair configuration (Fig. 1.3), which overcomes the difficult access situation.

An alternative strategy, especially in the home or office environment, is the use of a kitchen or office chair (Fig. 1.4). This provides a safe and comfortable means of negotiating corners and stairs, or other awkward obstacles.

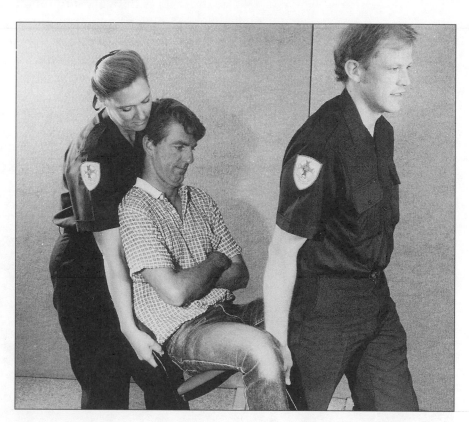

Fig. 1.4 Using the kitchen chair carry, the two rescuers can balance the load evenly and work together.

Indications
Patients with injury other than pelvic or lower limb problems. Moving an unconscious patient from a difficult position.

Precautions
Ensure that the chair is sturdy and not too heavy. If the move involves carrying down stairs, make sure the patient's arms are secure to prevent the patient from grabbing at objects during the manoeuvre.

The 'stretcher chair' requires assembly into the chair configuration before proceeding to the patient's location. Make certain that the locking devices are secure and restraining straps are positioned.

| **TASK** | Move a patient using a carry chair | 243 |

Stretchers

There are many types of stretchers used in ambulances. The most widely used are those comprising a stretcher and trolley, some of which are detachable (Fig. 1.5). The trolley is adjustable through a range of heights, improving safe handling. It is vital to spend some time becoming familiar with the adjustments to maximise efficient use and safety.

The stretcher is designed to fold into several positions, which will facilitate good patient management, e.g., head elevation to afford a suitable posture to assist breathing, or foot elevation to promote autoinfusion in shock management. The ability to detach the stretcher from the trolley increases its versatility in confined spaces and the carry chair configuration is a valuable asset for patient movement in the narrow passages of houses and in stair-wells.

TASKS		
1.	Lift a patient by the fore and aft method	240
2.	Place a patient on an ambulance stretcher	241
3.	Load a stretcher into an ambulance	242
4.	Unload a stretcher from an ambulance	242

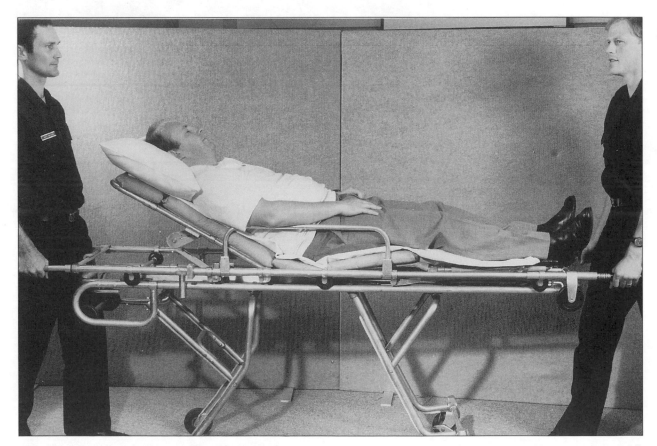

Fig. 1.5 The Ferno-Washington stretcher in use. The stretcher has been adjusted for patient comfort, and the trolley adjusted down one notch for stability while being moved.

ENVIRONMENTAL HAZARDS

1

Aim

To develop an appreciation of the hazards encountered in pre-hospital care and an understanding of prevention of personal injury and contamination

Learning plan

1. Read the text information
2. Develop a personal 'drill' for the approach to patient care

Pre-hospital care, as with all emergency service responses, exposes emergency personnel to many hazards. In the road crash incident there are physical hazards to note and avoid—the broken glass, jagged metal, petrol leaking from a ruptured tank and so on. However, there are other hazards which may not be immediately obvious—toxic fumes from chemicals, confined spaces where the air is unsafe, and cables cleverly hidden inside the power pole.

> **STOP AND LOOK FOR HAZARDS AT THE SCENE BEFORE COMMITTING YOURSELF—IT MAY MEAN YOUR LIFE**

(Chapters 2 and 8 discuss these problems in more detail.)

INFECTION

An area of potential hazard which has received much publicity in recent times is infection, especially hepatitis B and Acquired Immune Deficiency Syndrome (AIDS). The management of trauma patients invariably means that the ambulance officer will come into contact with a patient's blood or body fluids. Accidental cuts to fingers or hands from sharp objects at the scene raises the risk of 'blood to blood' contact.

Hepatitis B (HBV) is one of the major infectious diseases in the world. It is probably the most common cause of chronic liver disease and a cause of fatal malignancies (primary hepatocellular carcinoma (PHC)). HBV is recognised as a significant occupational hazard among health care personnel.

Transmission of hepatitis B is predominantly through contact with infected blood or blood products but the virus is also present in other body fluids.

Intravenous drug abusers, who share needles with other addicts, may readily acquire the disease. However, the risk of contamination is not restricted to only these recognised social behavioural groups. Care must be taken in the management of all patient contacts.

Acquired Immune Deficiency Syndrome (AIDS) is caused by a virus which was first discovered in 1983. It is now universally known as human immunodeficiency virus (HIV). The most common mode of transmission of HIV is through sexual intercourse. However, infected blood and blood products raises a significant risk in the emergency environment, where blood-to-blood contact is a likely event. Accidental cuts to fingers or hands from sharp objects or needles contaminated with the patient's blood, may expose the ambulance officer to the virus.

> **ALWAYS USE GLOVES WHEN PATIENT CONTACT MAY INVOLVE BLOOD OR BODY FLUIDS. THIS IS A VITAL ELEMENT OF THE PREVENTIVE CODE OF PRACTICE**

There is no evidence to date that suggests the virus is spread by saliva or social contact. The use of expired air resuscitation does not appear to place the rescuer at risk to HIV. The approach to patient care, when dealing with any possible infective contamination, including AIDS, is common sense. Use protective equipment and minimise personal contact with the patient. The wearing of masks and gowns, when transporting patients with infectious diseases, should be considered and advice sought from the requesting medical officer prior to transport.

Minimise the risk of infection—wear protective garments where necessary.

If despite the precautions taken, contamination with body fluids from an HBV or HIV carrier does occur, wash the area thoroughly with soap and water. If the skin is intact, avoid scrubbing to prevent blood stimulation in the skin, which may increase the risk of contamination. However, if the skin is punctured by needle stick or other sharp injury, encourage bleeding to reduce the potential for viral entry. Contamination to the eyes or mouth requires wash out with copious amounts of water. Eye irrigation with a sterile eye wash solution is preferable.

The incident reporting procedure and documentation should be completed and the ambulance service medical officer, or where established, the occupational health team should be notified.

The maintenance of a clean environment in the ambulance is important, from both the patient and crew points of view. The transfer of infection, especially in trauma patients with open wounds, is a significant risk if the patient compartment is not cleaned appropriately. Get into the healthy habit of cleaning the interior of the ambulance immediately after a case and leave the ambulance open and in sunlight whenever possible. Fresh air and sunlight are natural cleansing agents.

Clean the stretcher frame and mattress regularly to remove dirt and other contaminants and, of course, always dress the stretcher with fresh linen after each case.

Personal hygiene is paramount. Your own health is an important element in resisting infections to which you will be frequently exposed. Always have a change of clothing available in your locker at the ambulance station in case of clothing becoming soiled on the job.

Always follow local disinfecting policies.

DEALING WITH JOB DEMANDS

Aim

To develop an understanding of the stress process and identify coping behaviours

Learning plan

1. **Read the text information**
2. **Practise talking about events**

The very act of being alive places demands on people. These demands are created by families, friends and work. Usually we have little difficulty in coping with or meeting these demands and in fact they can be quite exhilarating, leading to a degree of satisfaction.

In a caring profession such as ambulance work, we spend a considerable portion of our time dealing with the crises of other individuals and families, involving both physical care and emotional support. By the very nature of this task, some circumstances, such as horrific road crashes involving death and mutilation, will produce some emotional impact on the ambulance officer.

Most student ambulance officers have strong doubts about their ability to cope with certain aspects of the job when they first join the service. If you have doubts about your ability to cope, one thing is certain—you are not alone. It is something that happens to all of us. However, if you have an understanding of what is happening to you when you experience stress, then you have a greater chance of coping with that stress.

THE STRESS PROCESS

Stress *events* are the things that happen to you, and may be real or imagined, the effects being equally disruptive. During your career, you will experience many events that will have some impact on you. It is not always a single incident that produces the overwhelming stress response, nor is it always a major incident. Often we are affected by an accumulation of experiences which we link together in our minds. Naturally, an incident, such as a plane crash or multiple vehicle road crash, does produce critical stress levels in some people, but the responses are not necessarily immediate.

The *thought process* of the stress picture is what you think about the event, making judgements about whether you will or will not cope with the event. This thought process can lead to behaviour, emotion and physiological changes.

Behaviour is what you do about the event, the action taken, usually in one of two ways—you deal with it or avoid it. In the emergency environment you cannot avoid the event, and the training undertaken enables you to respond effectively in most situations. However, the thought process after the event may cause you to doubt your ability to cope again and lead to avoidance through absenteeism or even contemplating a change of employment.

Emotion is how you feel about the event, or the feelings which result from thinking about the event. You might feel angry, disappointed or guilty if you think that you could not or did not deal with the event properly. However, you might have positive feelings about the event if you handled it well—feelings of satisfaction or even elation.

Changes in physiology are what happens in your body as a result of what you think about an event. Mostly, these changes are associated with preparing your body for action, such as increases in heart rate and blood pressure, blood flow to muscles, increased breathing and perspiration. Of course if you think that no action is required, then there may be no physiological changes in your body.

It is important to note that the three responses (behaviour, emotions and physiological changes) result from the thoughts about the event. If you have some understanding of the stress process, then intervention is possible.

INTERVENING IN THE STRESS PROCESS

The view that stress is a sign of weakness or unsuitability for emergency work is not now widely held. The need for developing coping skills and providing counselling processes for emergency workers has been recognised and, in many services, has been established. In the ambulance environment, much can be achieved by peer support and debriefing tasks as early as possible after the event.

Discuss your feelings about the event with your crew partner—he or she is probably experiencing similar emotions.

Families and friends are often neglected as a source of support. Ambulance officers tend not to discuss their experiences at home because of the nature of the tasks. However, sharing anxieties about the job may not only help to resolve your feelings, but reduce personal conflicts which may occur because of your changed behaviour from the experience.

Discuss your feelings about events with your family—don't isolate yourself.

The physiological response to stress not only involves the features of raised pulse and blood pressure, but often many people experience prolonged muscle tension, lower back pain or clenched teeth and aching in the jaw. This stress can be relieved by *relaxation techniques*. It may seem obvious, but consciously relaxing can have a positive effect on the negative physiological responses to stress, especially those of long duration.

Relaxation involves getting into a comfortable position and concentrating on muscle groups in your body. Start at the feet and gradually work up your body, tensing each part for about 5 seconds and then relaxing. When you have worked up to your head, relax your whole body as much as you can for about 10 minutes. Try to imagine, as vividly as possible, a scene that is relaxing for you. When you have finished, open your eyes and get up slowly.

Relaxation is a skill which can be learnt and you improve with practice. There are many audio tape programmes which you may find helpful, or you might consider joining a relaxation class.

Stress is manifested in many different ways in all of us. If we take the time to identify the effect and exercise coping mechanisms, the outcomes can be positive and worthwhile.

DRIVING AN EMERGENCY VEHICLE

Aim

To develop an awareness of defensive driving principles applied to patient care transport

Learning plan

1. Read the text information
2. Check your local road regulations for the exemptions pertaining to emergency vehicles
3. Check your service's policies for any procedures relating to emergency vehicle operations
4. Practise the defensive driving principles in your own car

The operation of an emergency vehicle is vastly different from the way in which a passenger vehicle is driven by most drivers in the community. An ambulance conveying an injured or sick patient must provide a smooth ride to reduce the effects of travel, and of equal importance, a stable patient care platform upon which patient care may be safely continued during transit.

Normal functions of braking, acceleration and cornering are vital skills to be developed to reduce the tendency to throw the passengers against the restraints in the vehicle. A patient who is ill and transported on a stretcher in the patient compartment may be adversely affected by sway and other harsh movements.

Responding to an emergency call enables the ambulance officer to exercise the *privileges* granted to emergency vehicles under road traffic legislation.

Always remember traffic legislation gives emergency vehicles privileges, not rights.

Emergency responses require the use of both audible and visual warning devices. This does not necessarily mean that all road users will be aware of the approach and that the way is clear to proceed. Modern passenger vehicles are equipped with air conditioners, sophisticated radios and other devices, which may restrict the driver from hearing the siren. In fact many road users drive with 'tunnel vision' and are not aware of traffic behind their vehicle.

> **ALWAYS TAKE CARE COMING UP BEHIND TRAFFIC AND IF IN DOUBT, HANG BACK**

The skills in driving an emergency vehicle must be practised as frequently as possible, even in the car while driving to and from work. The system of car control is not different and can be applied to all vehicles.

The most significant aspect of driving is attitude. Aggressive behaviour leads to errors and disaster. Likewise, the use of high speed must be carefully considered. In the built up areas of cities and towns, speed will not necessarily get the ambulance to the scene more quickly. A slower approach may mean that there are fewer occasions when the passage to the scene is obstructed and the trip therefore is smoother. If the journey is stressful, the efficiency of patient care on arrival may be less than desirable.

Spend some time becoming familiar with the local environment so that you develop an understanding of the congested areas, best routes to take and the nature of the road surfaces.

Remember, you have a responsibility to your crew partner, the patient, other road users, and importantly, yourself.

MEDICO-LEGAL CONSIDERATIONS

Aim

To develop an understanding of the law as it affects pre-hospital patient care

Learning plan

1. Read the text information
2. Check your service's policies and protocols for the scope of practice and the restrictions imposed
3. Supplement your reading with the Coroner's Act

The legal systems in all countries which were settled by English speaking people, have their origins in English law and are similar. Ambulance services operate under statutory authority, given by an Act of Parliament. The provisions hold the service accountable and responsible for the actions of the individual officer, provided that an incident is not the result of negligence or a breach of civil or criminal law. The Act allows an ambulance officer to operate as a 'limited agent' for the service's medical officer, with regard to the use of invasive procedures and pharmacological substances. This authority to act is specified in protocols and defined procedures, which identify the *scope of practice*. Departure from the protocols and defined procedures of the service may result in legal action against the individual, either by the patient (or family) or following a coronial enquiry, although this is rare.

Liability for negligence results from

- causing injury to a patient
- failure to act, when the individual has a duty to act
- failure to act appropriately which causes injury.

Unlike the police officer, who may act whether on duty or off duty, the ambulance officer may only operate within the scope of ambulance practice while engaged on a rostered duty. Once off duty, the scope of practice is limited to first aid—what might be expected of any citizen. The use of pharmacological substances (e.g., analgesics) or operational protocols and procedures is illegal off duty.

The ambulance service and its officers are required to respond to all calls for assistance. The execution of this duty to act requires the *consent* of the patient to accept the care and transport provided. In most circumstances the ambulance officer is providing basic care in response to a call, and the question of consent does not arise. However, the administration of drugs or any task that requires physical contact with the patient, should be consented to by the patient before commencement. Consent is equally effective at law in written, oral and implied forms. Implied refers to events in which the patient is unconscious or unable to act rationally and requires emergency care, justifying treatment in the absence of verbal or written consent. The management of children, especially where administration of drugs is required, should be with the consent of a parent.

The law provides the individual with the right to freedom of movement. The transport of a patient by ambulance, without the consent of the patient, thus restricting the individual's right of free movement, may bring about an action of *false imprisonment*. However, in the case of confinement under the mental health legislation, the ambulance officer is protected, provided that the documentation is complete and signed by an attending physician or other person authorised under the Act.

The *restraint* of patients, by mechanical means, applies to circumstances specified by law:

- to prevent personal injury or injury to other persons
- to prevent persistent destruction of property
- for the purposes of administering treatment.

The provisions of restraint, relevant to pre-hospital care, are those under the mental health legislation. Only those patients who have been referred to a psychiatric centre by an attending physician or other authorised person, who has duly completed the required documentation, can be legally restrained.

The laws covering ambulance practice, mental health patients and pre-hospital care vary to some extent from country to country, and from State to State in Australia. The ambulance officer should be acquainted with the relevant Acts and conditions under which the ambulance service operates.

FURTHER READING

Beverley P et al 1987 ABC of AIDS. British Medical Journal, London
Jayson M 1981 Back pain, the facts. Oxford University Press, London
McNab F 1985 Coping. Hill Of Content, Melbourne
Montgomery R 1985 Coping with stress. Pitman, Melbourne
Pelosi A, Gleeson M 1988 Illustrated transfer techniques for disabled people. Churchill Livingstone, Melbourne

CHAPTER 2
Getting started

The approach to an incident requires a systematic analysis of events and actions to manage the priorities of patient care beginning with life threatening events. This preliminary information puts together the basis upon which clinical problems can be managed in the pre-hospital care environment.

Topics covered

Primary survey
Vital signs survey
Secondary survey
Patient care records

Pre-hospital care is today very much a specialised component of the modern health care system. It draws its procedures and protocols from the essentials of the hospital emergency and intensive care departments. To make all this happen smoothly and efficiently, in an environment which has limited resources, a structured approach is needed. This enables data to be collected in a methodical manner to allow sound decision making and the instigation of appropriate care, without unnecessary delay at the scene of an incident.

As we go further into emergency care and the so-called 'advanced life support' skills, it is vital that a solid foundation is prepared upon which the new technology can be used.

PRIMARY SURVEY

Aim

To develop a systematic approach to dealing with life threatening problems

Learning plan

1. Read the text information and check your understanding using the knowledge check
2. Practise the steps of the primary survey using the flowchart as a guide
3. Practise the life essential skills using the skills guides as a reference check

Approaching any incident involves prioritising actions, beginning with those which will deal with life threatening events. This first part of the approach is the primary survey, focussing attention on the immediate intervention required to prevent death.

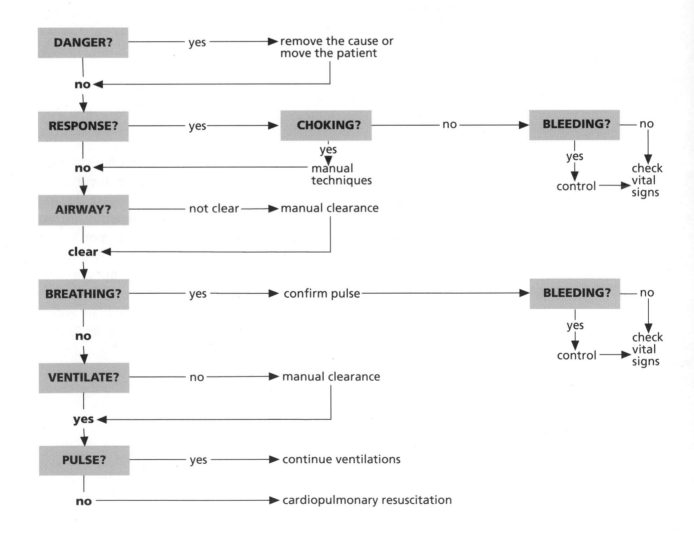

Fig. 2.1 The primary survey flowchart.

Using the flowchart (Fig. 2.1), the steps are:

DANGER?

This is the first priority to ensure the safety of the ambulance officer, the patient(s) and bystanders.

Look for hazards at the scene. There may be broken glass, unstable structures, smoke, fire, fumes, or broken electrical power lines and appliances.

Care must be exercised as many hazards are not immediately obvious.

Options: Remove the cause—for example, clear loose debris, extinguish the fire, switch off the power—or move the patient. In circumstances where the hazard cannot be safely and quickly managed or where access or control is not possible, *do not proceed* but seek the assistance of other combating authorities.

RESPONSE?

Does the patient respond to shout and shake?

The purpose of this step is to establish if the patient is conscious or unconscious. If unconscious, the immediate concern is the potential loss of airway control. At this time the focus is only directed towards whether the patient is reacting to normal stimulus. Ask 'Can you hear me?', 'Open your eyes', 'What is your name?' Grasp the patient's shoulders and shake gently.

CHOKING?

Is the patient choking?

Acute obstruction of the upper airway, either partial or complete, may cause altered consciousness and lead to respiratory arrest unless prompt action is taken. The effects of airway obstruction will depend on the degree of obstruction and the subsequent adequacy or inadequacy of air exchange. If air exchange is inadequate the patient may be coughing violently with noisy breathing. If air exchange is inadequate, the patient may panic, clutch the throat and show acute distress. This may be followed rapidly by cyanosis and altered consciousness. If the patient can speak and breathe, encourage coughing which may help dislodge the foreign material. If the patient is unable to speak or breathe, a range of manual techniques are available to attempt removal—gravity and finger probing, back blows and abdominal thrusts—and all should be utilised. If the patient has a wheeze following successful relief of an obstruction, this may suggest partial obstruction requiring medical intervention.

AIRWAY?

Does the patient have a clear airway?

This is the most significant priority in the assessment and management of the unconscious patient. If the airway is not clear and open, the patient is at grave risk. Management of the airway can be achieved by the *head tilt/jaw support* method. However, if copious amounts of fluid are obvious on inspection, the airway should be cleared by turning the patient on to one side.

BREATHING?

Is the patient breathing spontaneously?

This is the second significant priority in eliminating life threat to the unconscious patient. The only concern at this stage of management is whether air is moving freely in and out. Look for chest/abdominal movements. Listen for air moving in and out (noise will indicate other airway problems). Feel for air against your cheek while listening.

If the patient is breathing, confirm the pulse and check for external bleeding. At this stage, internal or concealed bleeding is not considered.

If the patient is not breathing, ventilate.

VENTILATE?

Can the patient be ventilated?

Time is vital. If the patient is not breathing, ventilation must be commenced immediately. Place the patient flat on the back (supine) with the airway maintained. Ventilation may be achieved by the expired air resuscitation method (EAR) or by the use of an oxygen powered or mechanical ventilator. Give five* full breaths in rapid succession. If ventilation cannot be achieved, (that is, no air entering no rise and fall of the patient's chest/abdomen), apply abdominal thrusts and re-check the airway. If further attempts fail to relieve the obstruction, attempt to ventilate by forceful pressure. This may dislodge the obstruction and move it into one side of the lungs, enabling partial ventilation.

PULSE?

Does the patient have a pulse?

This is the last sequential step in eliminating the life threat to the patient. The pulse assessment is brief, to confirm whether there is cardiac output. Further evaluation of rate, rhythm and strength is performed in the vital signs survey. The pulse is assessed by palpating

---

* In some resuscitation protocols, two initial ventilations are recommended.

the carotid artery. If the pulse is present, but breathing is absent, continue ventilations. However, if the pulse is absent, cardiopulmonary resuscitation (CPR) must be commenced immediately.

BLEEDING (EXTERNAL)?

Is there any evidence of major external bleeding?

A search for obvious bleeding is the final check in eliminating life threat problems and is performed after ensuring that the airway is clear, the patient is breathing, and the pulse is present. This is a quick survey to identify significant external bleeding which constitutes a life threat. Check the patient quickly from head to toes by look and feel. Any significant bleeding must be managed immediately by direct pressure, elevation, and the application of a pressure bandage.

Remember to check under the clothing. Thick garments may hide the evidence of bleeding and show little or no sign of underlying penetrating injury.

ABOUT AIRWAY MANAGEMENT

In this life threat phase, upper airway obstruction is the most common problem encountered. The airway will be discussed in more detail in Chapter 5, but a quick look inside the mouth will help orientation.

The most obvious structure observed, other than the teeth, is the tongue. If we observe the back (posterior) of the tongue, we notice that it is hinged to the lower jaw (mandible). In a conscious individual, muscles keep the jaw, and hence the tongue, in a normal position which affords a clear air pathway to the lungs. But if the patient is unconscious, the muscles relax, allowing the jaw to fall back (if the patient is on the back) and carry the tongue with it. Therefore, the tongue blocks the airway, stopping air entry, without which we cannot survive.

Clearing tongue obstruction then is a simple matter of manipulating the jaw. Tilting the head backwards and supporting the lower jaw in most cases will reduce the obstruction (Fig. 2.2 on page 24). Occasionally, thrusting the mandible at the angle of the jaw may be necessary. Placing the patient in a stable side position will engage the help of gravity in keeping the jaw, and hence the tongue, forward.

The use of an oropharyngeal airway will reduce the tendency to tongue obstruction and assist in maintaining an air pathway, but *will not* provide protection from fluids or other obstructions. Gravity will help to drain fluids from the airway. Normal secretions, blood and vomitus require rapid removal and in most cases, this can be easily achieved by turning the patient into a stable side position—especially in the event of copious fluids. Loose materials and solid debris must be manually removed by 'sweeping' the mouth. This is achieved by using the index and middle fingers of one *gloved* hand, inserted into one side

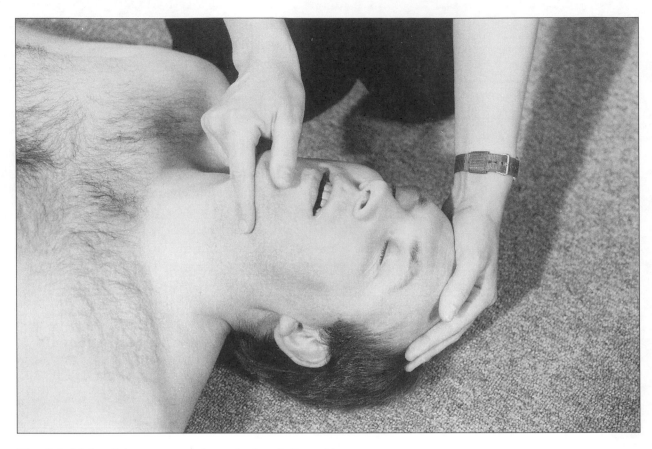

Fig. 2.2 Maintaining an open airway by head tilt and jaw support.

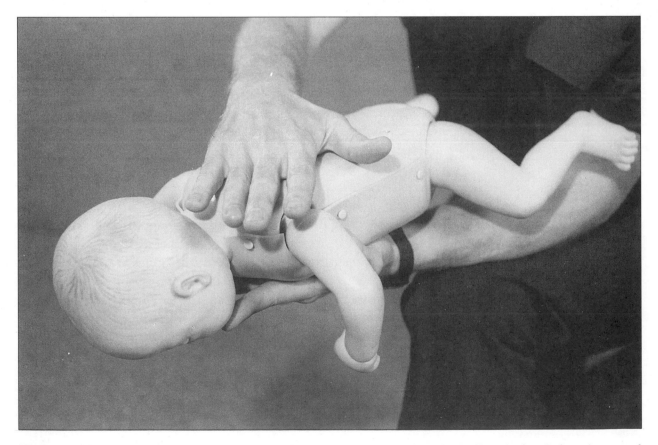

Fig. 2.3 When administering back blows to infants, support the patient, including the head, face down and strike the back firmly with the palm of one hand.

of the mouth and with a sweeping action, clearing debris out of the mouth. Mechanical suction devices are effective in the removal of fluids only, but as was mentioned earlier, a stable side posture, which enlists the aid of gravity, is more immediately effective, especially in the removal of copious fluid volumes.

Less common, but indeed not rare, is obstruction by a foreign body. Broken teeth or dentures may create this problem in situations involving facial trauma. Inhaled objects—for example, peanuts, marbles, buttons and coins—are frequent crises in children. A significant cause of foreign body obstruction in adults is food particles, especially small bones.

The immediate care involves gravity and back blows (Fig. 2.3) and in circumstances where the patient does not respond and ventilation attempts fail, the alternative method is abdominal thrusts (Fig. 2.4).

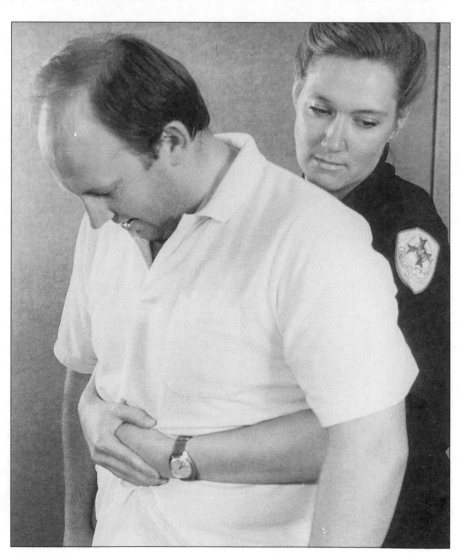

Fig. 2.4 Abdominal thrusts are a method of clearing airway obstruction in adults.

In 1974, Heimlich described a manoeuvre, which consisted of upward thrusts applied forcefully with the fist over the epigastrium and directed towards the diaphragm. While scientific evidence to support and prove the efficacy of abdominal thrusts is limited, there is sufficient anecdotal evidence to suggest that the manoeuvre should be considered as one of a range of options in the management of foreign body obstruction.

Obstruction may be caused by swelling of the tissues of the upper airway. This may be due to an allergic reaction to food, medications, or toxins (e.g., insect stings). Airway burns, following inhalation of hot gases or the fumes of corrosive substances and chemicals, result in mucosal swelling (angio-oedema). This is characterised by harsh whistling breathing (stridor). Airway burns and potential obstruction should be suspected in circumstances where the patient presents with facial burns and singed hair. (Burn injuries are considered in more detail in Chapter 6.) The third group of predisposing factors resulting in obstruction due to swelling is infection—commonly croup (and epiglottitis, although a less frequent incident) in children.

CARDIOPULMONARY RESUSCITATION

The aim of the primary survey, the subject of this part of the chapter, is to identify and eliminate life threatening events. Having dealt with the airway, the first significant priority, the next considerations are non-breathing and pulselessness. Cardiorespiratory arrest is the sudden and unexpected cessation of circulation and respiration.

During the past 25-30 years, many advances in life support have occurred and old techniques have been refashioned to provide new systems in resuscitation. In the 1950s Elam proved the superiority of exhaled air ventilation over manual breathing methods (Silvesters and Holger-Neilson) and since that time the 'mouth to mouth' method has been employed. A research team led by Kouwenhaven rediscovered and developed external cardiac compression in the 1960s, based on the Boehm and Schiffs open chest cardiac resuscitation techniques from the 19th century. In the early 1960s, expired air resuscitation and external cardiac compression were combined to create cardiopulmonary resuscitation (CPR). The concept of CPR has been adopted worldwide with community based training programmes as well as its use in emergency services and hospitals.

The success of CPR depends heavily on perfection of techniques and the early initiation of the procedure in the life threat incident. The brain is the most sensitive and important organ of the human body. After 3-6 minutes of cessation of heart/lung function, irreversible changes occur at the cellular level. Restoration of the oxygenation system must be commenced within this time interval if the patient is to survive. Cardiorespiratory arrest may result from:

1. Hypoxia (low oxygen)
   - due to reduced oxygen in the atmosphere (e.g., a smoke filled room)
   - due to airway obstruction (e.g., tongue, inhaled vomitus, foreign bodies)
   - through respiratory centre depression due to poisons, drugs or head injury
   - due to respiratory mechanism damage (injury to the chest wall
   - because of lung injury or disease (e.g., pneumothorax, drowning or pulmonary oedema)
   - due to severe blood loss (hypovolaemia).
2. Cardiovascular disturbance
   - due to inadequate heart function (e.g., acute myocardial infarction—(AMI))
   - through disruption of heart function (e.g., electrocution).

These causes will be explored more completely later, but for now, let's concentrate on the essential skills.

> The recognition of cardiorespiratory arrest consists of three key observations:
> 1. No response
> 2. Absence of respirations
> 3. Absence of carotid pulse

The patient may also present with extreme pallor (cyanosis may be present) and fixed, dilated pupils. The immediate action is firstly to *recognise* the problem, then *provide artificial ventilation* and *artificial circulation*.

Artificial ventilation

The mouth to mouth method or ventilation equipment may be used. In the ambulance environment, ventilation equipment is available. However, it is important to develop skills in a variety of approaches—with and without equipment.

In recent times, much has been written about the risks of contracting diseases—in particular hepatitis B and AIDS. The application of the mouth to mouth method of resuscitation, as with all patient contact procedures, raises the risks of disease transfer. However, apart from blood-to-blood contact, there is low risk from saliva contact and assistance should not be withheld. Face shields are widely available to minimise the disease problem and if there is some concern about the possibility of contamination, a face mask can be used.

Artificial circulation

First, the position of the heart muscle must be correctly located. It lies behind the lower half of the sternum, with the apex to the left, in the 5th intercostal space in the mid-clavicular line. The base lies slightly to the right of the sternum, from the level of the 3rd—6th costal cartilage (Fig. 2.5 on page 28).

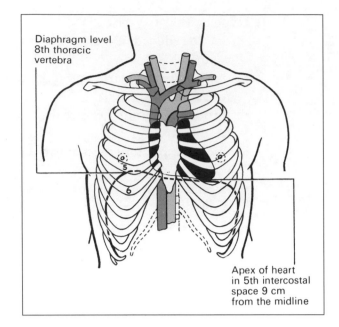

Diaphragm level
8th thoracic
vertebra

Apex of heart
in 5th intercostal
space 9 cm
from the midline

Fig. 2.5 The position of the heart in the thorax.
(Reproduced with permission from Wilson K J W 1990 Ross & Wilson: Anatomy and physiology in health and illness, 7th edition. Churchill Livingstone, Edinburgh)

> The position of the hands during cardiac compression is a critical factor:
> - TOO HIGH = INEFFECTIVE
> - TOO LOW = INEFFECTIVE
>   and risk of gross damage to the liver

There are two principal methods for locating the correct compression point. The 'caliper' method (Fig. 2.6) locates the midpoint of the sternum and the heel of the lower hand is placed so that the thumbs are touching. The alternative method is achieved by locating the lower end of the sternum (xyphisternum) and placing two fingers to cover the bony prominence. The lower hand is then positioned above the fingers. It matters not which method is used. The critical point is that the hands are located on the lower half of the sternum, immediately over the heart.

The compression technique requires the heel of the hand to remain in contact with the patient's chest constantly during compressions. Moving from the correct position may cause damage to the chest wall. Vertical pressure is applied to a depth of 4-5cm, and released to allow the chest to return to its normal position, creating a 50/50 pressure cycle.

In a single rescuer incident, the ratio of compressions to ventilations is **15:2**—that is, 15 external cardiac compressions followed by 2 lung inflations in rapid succession. This cycle should be sustained at a frequency of 4-5 cycles per minute, the number of cycles per minute being more important than the rate of compression.

> CPR—Single rescuer
> Ratio 15:2

Fig. 2.6 How to place the hands when locating the compression point for cardiac compression using the 3-step caliper method.

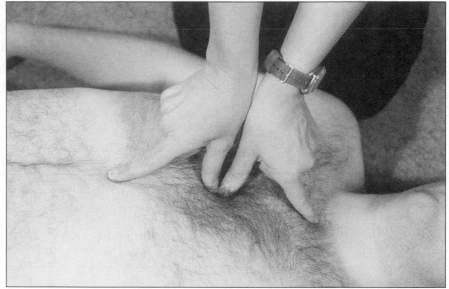
a

a. Dividing the sternum using finger and thumb to locate the midpoint.

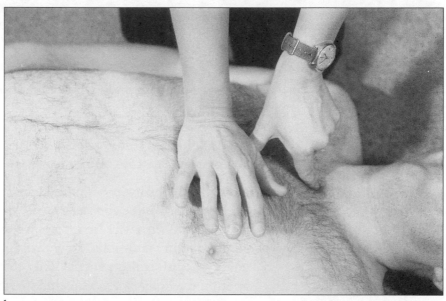
b

b. Placing the hand below the midpoint of the sternum thumb to thumb.

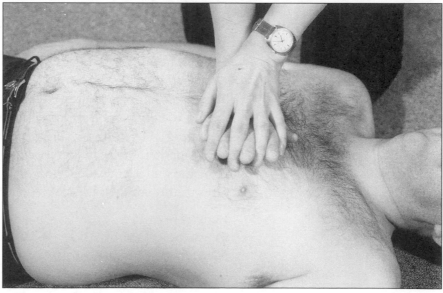
c

c. Final interlocked position of both hands for compression.

In a two-rescuer incident, CPR is performed at a ratio of **5:1**—that is, 5 external cardiac compressions, with 1 lung inflation interposed between each 5th and 1st compressions. The cycles should be sustained at a rate of 12-15 per minute. This 'team' rescue is more efficient, because there is no interruption to external cardiac compression.

CPR—Two rescuers
Ratio 5:1

TASKS

VITAL SIGNS SURVEY

Aim

To develop a base upon which time critical decisions are made

Learning plan

1. **Read the text information**
2. **Complete the case history exercise**

Now that the problems of immediate life threat have been dealt with, the next phase of the approach is the vital signs survey. This focuses on the question: 'How sick is the patient?' The survey provides a *whole body* clinical picture and is the only means in the field to determine what is going on inside the patient. This total picture enables judgement about the *urgency of treatment* and whether to continue on-site care or consider early transport to the emergency department; that is, 'Is the patient *time critical?*'

The vital signs survey is a specified series of important observations, which can be quickly made, repeated, and enable an objective assessment about the patient's *general* condition. It helps to confirm that the patient who 'looks sick', is 'indeed sick'. The information gained enables informed judgements about the whole patient and the effect the incident is having on the patient (whether improving or deteriorating). The survey consists of three elements which, when viewed together, help in determining the time critical patient or whether the patient may be seriously ill, although appearing well now. Using a trauma model, the elements are:

- Pattern of injury
- Physiological status
- Mechanism of injury.

However, the survey can be applied equally to the ill patient. (See Fig. 2.7)

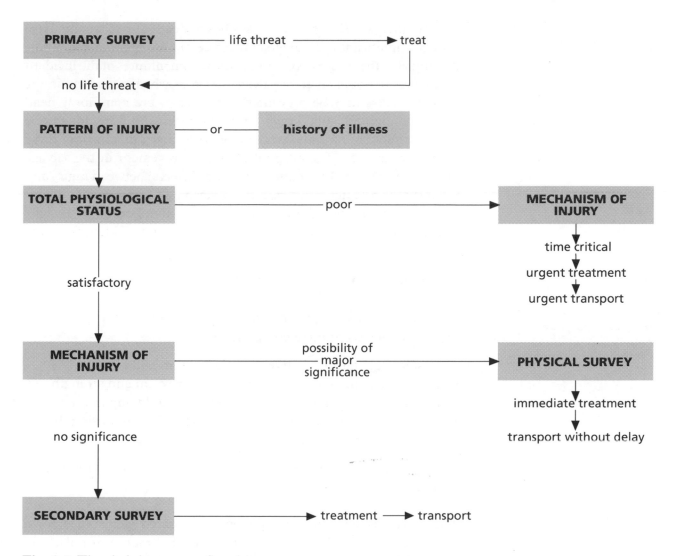

Fig. 2.7 The vital signs survey flowchart.

PATTERN OF INJURY

The pattern of injury helps in directing the rescuer to potential injuries in various situations. Think about a driver of a car in a head-on collision who is not wearing a seatbelt. Certain incidents classically cause a certain pattern of injury and these injuries should be regarded as being present until proven otherwise.

However, of significance is the type and location of major injury patterns. There are two basic injury patterns to consider involving the head, neck, chest, abdomen or pelvis:

- Penetrating injuries
- Blunt injuries.

The injury pattern is of greater significance if it involves two or more of the above regions or two or more proximal long bone fractures.

While the patterns of injury are not true vital signs, they can be used effectively in conjunction with physiological data to determine the potential salvageability of trauma patients and therefore those who are time critical.

Over the past 20 years, many studies of death due to trauma have shown a significant percentage of these deaths are preventable. While it is arguable that those patients who die within minutes of the incident occurring are not likely to be salvaged, deaths which occur within the first few hours may be prevented. The causes are commonly head injury, lung injury, solid organ damage (spleen and liver) long bone and multiple trauma with severe blood loss. Given that most of these deaths occur in the pre-hospital phase, improvement in the salvage rate may be achieved by reducing the time interval between injury and the institution of definitive care in the hospital setting.

If we accept that there is a significant number of potentially salvageable patients, then the next question is how to identify them.

PHYSIOLOGICAL STATUS

Physiological status is the objective, clinical element of the vital signs survey. It consists of three components:

- Respiratory status—a survey of rate, rhythm and effort
- Perfusion status—a survey of pulse rate, rhythm and strength, blood pressure, capillary refill, skin colour and temperature
- Conscious status—a survey of neurological function using the Glasgow Coma Scale.

(Each of the components are explored in detail in the following clinical chapters.)

The data collected in each component is compared against the known normal physiological values (e.g., the accepted ranges of pulse and respiratory rates). The first set of physiological data serves two purposes:

- Immediate evidence of changed homeostasis which requires urgent management
- A baseline against which further data may be compared to judge improvement or deterioration.

Over recent years, a number of trauma severity scales and scores have been developed which attempt to quantify physiological data in a numeric a form. The object is to identify the salvageable patient and simplify decision making in both the pre-hospital environment and the hospital emergency department. To date, there is little agreement about the best scale, and apart from the Glasgow Coma Scale, there is little uniformity of use within emergency medicine. Numerical values are of no significance unless there is uniform use in the emergency medical system.

The charting of physiological status is one of the most important functions to be carried out in the field, as it not only enables decisions to be made on-site, but provides a beginning point for the emergency department on which further definitive care can be based. Consider the patient who was the driver of a motor vehicle, not wearing a seatbelt and involved in a collision. On initial examination, the pattern of injury shows no major injury of the type described earlier. The physiological status at this time is acceptable. But, is the patient likely to deteriorate?

MECHANISM OF INJURY

The guidelines for determining potential injury relate to an assessment of the mechanism of injury and the history of:

- What happened in the incident?
- What happened to the patient in the incident?

The assessment of potential injury forces us to think of the internal organs—what injury might they have sustained, but as yet is not apparent. The importance of this element of the survey is to identify possible internal injury, because once the patient deteriorates, as a result of internal injury, there is little that can be done in the pre-hospital setting. Such patients should be transported expeditiously, and in this sense, transport is treatment.

The concept of *time critical* patients refers also to patients, where some evidence from the mechanism of injury suggests that there is injury of major significance. Evidence from recent trauma studies suggests a golden hour—that is, patients with initially non-apparent or hidden injuries may be able to compensate and maintain a reasonable clinical and physiological status for an hour or so before deteriorating. Such potential disaster should be identified early and patients transported to the emergency department within this hour time frame.

The guidelines for the mechanism of blunt injuries, which may be of *major significance* are:

- Involvement in high speed (over 75 k.p.h.) collisions
- Pedestrians hit by vehicles travelling over 30 k.p.h
- Passengers who are thrown from vehicles by the collision
- Falls from heights over 6 metres.

TASK   Complete the case history   43

SECONDARY SURVEY

Aim

To develop a systematic approach to the physical assessment of the patient

Learning plan

1. Read the text information
2. Practise the nose-to-toes survey to develop your style

The final step in the approach to an incident is to answer the questions, 'What is the major presenting problem?' and 'What other problems are present?' This secondary survey indicates the specific treatment needed. Following the trauma theme of this chapter, the survey is a careful and thorough physical assessment of the body—the nose-to-toes surface check. There is often the tendency to move to the obvious and miss the more significant injury. A systematic approach ensures that *nothing* is *overlooked*. One systematic approach to consider is the nose-to-toes surface check (Fig. 2.8).

HEAD AND NECK

- Check the scalp for bleeding
- Check the skull for lumps or depressions
- Look for fluid discharge from the ears, nose or mouth (Fluid discharge from these openings may be an indicator of base of skull fracture.)
- Feel the neck gently for deformity.

BACK

- Feel carefully for obvious irregularities of the spine
- Feel for indications of bleeding.

CHEST WALL

- Look and feel for unnatural chest movement
- Feel gently for fractures
- Look for wounds.

ABDOMEN

- Look for discolouration, abrasions, open wounds
- Feel for rigidity or muscle spasm.

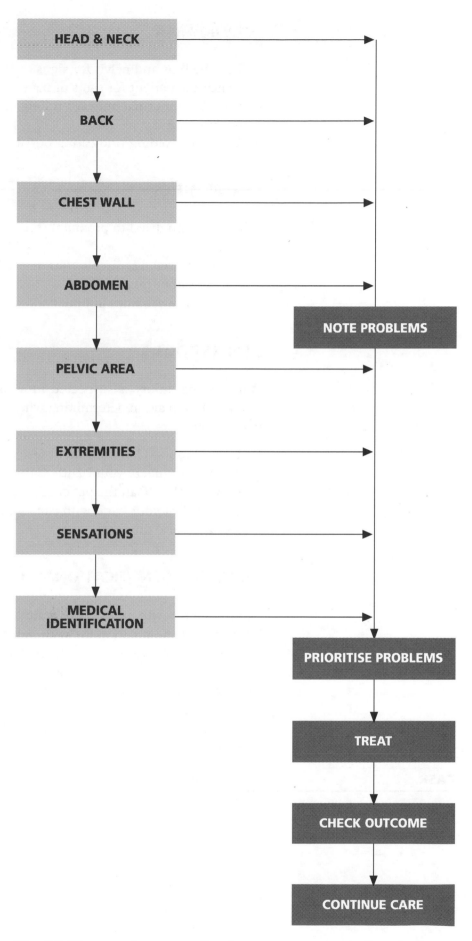

Fig. 2.8 The secondary survey flowchart; a nose to toes surface check.

PELVIC AREA

- Feel the hips and pelvis for signs of fracture
- Watch the patient for signs of pain
- Look for abnormal outward rolling of the legs (indicating possible hip injury)
- Check for voiding (indicating possible pelvic injury).

EXTREMITIES

- Check from distal to proximal (fingers to shoulder and toes to hips)
- Look for swelling, discolouration and bleeding
- Look for abnormal features
- Feel for irregularities in bones

SENSATIONS

Where spinal injury is suspected in a conscious patient, a series of quick tests will aid in determining whether paralysis is present and to what extent:

- Upper limbs—Can the patient feel your touch? Can the patient grasp and squeeze your hand? Can the patient move both limbs?
- Lower limbs—Can the patient feel your touch? Can the patient push against your hand with each foot? Can the patient move the toes and raise the leg?

MEDICAL IDENTIFICATION

Many people with potentially serious medical conditions wear a bracelet or pendant to assist with early identification of problems. Look for these, particularly when examining an unconscious patient. Contained within, or on the back is the primary medical problem, drug sensitivity and normally a contact number for further details.

Complete the systematic survey of the whole body *before* treating any injury found. When the survey is finished, prioritise the injuries in an order for treatment.

SUMMARY

The approach to an incident is a systematic analysis of the event, incorporating judgements and actions in a logically planned manner to ensure that all priorities are met and that adequate, relevant data are collected. The approach consists of the 3 phases of primary survey, vital signs survery and secondary survey.

1. The *primary survey*, focuses on life threat problems:

> Danger
> Response—Choking—Bleeding
> Airway
> Breathing—Bleeding
> Ventilate
> Pulse

2. The *vital signs survey*, is the data collecting and decision making phase concerning the critical patient:

> Pattern of injury + Physiological status + Mechanism of injury

3. The *secondary survey* is the full surface check to prioritise treatment and ensure that nothing is overlooked:

> Nose-to-toes surface check

While the description of this chapter has been a trauma model—which is conceptually easier to follow—the phases can be readily adapted to managing the ill patient. Likewise the secondary survey can be adapted to clinical investigation of specific illness problems, the subject of the following chapters.

2

PATIENT CARE RECORDS

Aim

To develop an understanding of the requirements for medical documentation and skill in completing pre-hospital patient care records

Learning plan

1. Read the text information
2. Check your service's patient care document to ensure that you are aware of the requirements
3. Complete a patient care record for each of the case history exercises in the clinical chapters using your service's patient care document

An essential element of the provision of health care is the recording of medical history and management. In pre-hospital care, this recording of data provides the first base line of evidence, which assists the emergency department and other critical care areas of the hospital to identify the urgent needs of the patient. If the record is incomplete or cannot be accurately interpreted, the outcome could be a delay in the provision of vital treatment. It should also be clearly understood that the ambulance record is admissible evidence in a court of law and, therefore, must be accurate in every detail.

The ambulance patient care record is a valuable source of information for the ambulance service. Not only is it the means by which patient accounts are prepared, but the record facilitates medical audit, training and statistical data gathering.

Patient care record designs vary considerably from service to service, so the emphasis in this text is in the recording of physiological data, history of the incident, findings made by the ambulance officer and the details of management.

PHYSIOLOGICAL DATA

The presentation of the patient's vital signs during care at the scene and subsequent transport provides a clear picture of physiological trends if it is arranged in a chart form (Fig.2.9 on pages 40–41). The Glasgow Coma Scale is commonly incorporated in most charts to provide a good record of the patient's conscious status, alongwith perfusion and respiratory status details. Improvement, stability or deterioration can be seen at a glance.

HISTORY OF THE INCIDENT

Relevant information about the incident is useful in determining the direction of investigations and appropriate treatments. In the trauma incident, information about impact velocity, the position of the patient and what happened in the event, may give valuable clues to potential injury patterns. This data can be displayed, especially in road crash incidents, by the use of a diagram of a motor vehicle (Fig. 2.9). The recording of relevant information in incidents of acute illness is often charted in a narrative-style form. This information should be arranged in a logical order, under suitable headings:

- Main presenting problem, which is the reason for the ambulance response to the incident. This should be written in general terms and not as a diagnosis, e.g., the main presenting problem in illness of cardiac origin is chest pain and shortness of breath
- Relevant past history, noting if the patient has had previous episodes and what medication the patient is currently taking
- On arrival, what was observed which might be relevant to the emergency department in understanding the incident, e.g., the attitude and position of the patient
- On examination, which is a brief description of relevant clinical information, from the examination of the patient. Avoid repeating the physiological data recorded in the chart format. The final component of the history section should include a statement of the initial assessment in problem terms, again not as a diagnosis. This may include a judgement of the time critical nature of the patient.

Body charts are used widely to illustrate the location of problem areas, such as the location of fractures or regions of pain and paralysis. While the body chart is a suitable adjunct to the record, it can become almost useless if it is cluttered with too much information. Restrict the recording of details on the chart to important findings and use a standard list of abbreviations.

MANAGEMENT

The last section of the patient care record documents the specific treatment given during the pre-hospital care phase. This should include all significant procedures and drugs, the time they were administered and the outcome of treatment.

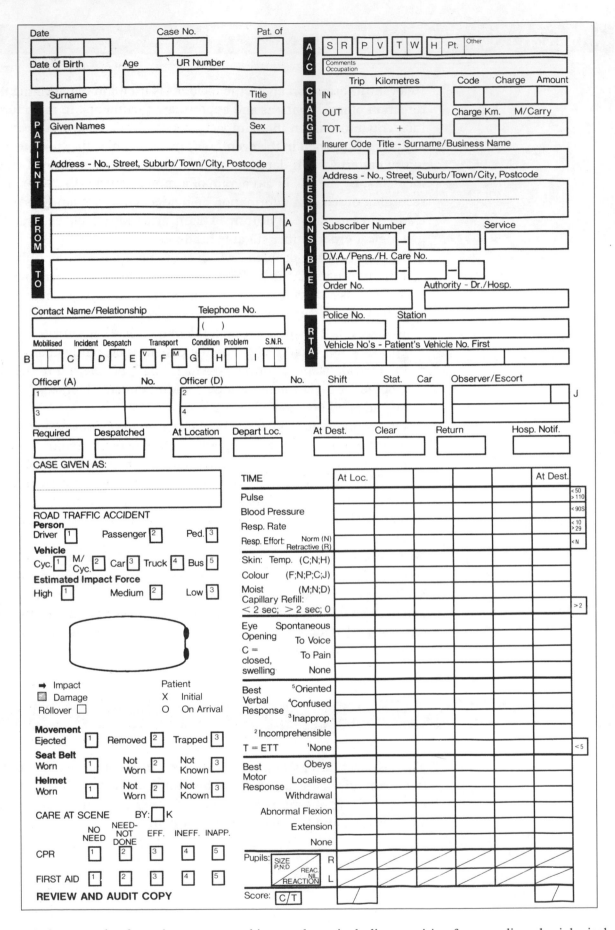

Fig. 2.9 An example of a patient care record in actual use, including provision for recording physiological data in chart form. (Reproduced with permission from the Victorian Ambulance Services Association.)

Main Presenting Problem (MP);   Relevant Past History (PHx);   Medication (Med𝗻);
History (Hx);   On arrival (O/A);   On Examination (O/E).

MP
PHx.
Med𝗻.
Hx.
O/A.
O/E.

INITIAL ASSESSMENT		Time Critical	Y	N
		Trauma Alert	Y	N

DOCTOR AT SCENE   No ☐   Yes ☐

REMOTE MEDICAL CONSULTATION   No ☐   Yes ☐

Dr's Name/Hosp. or Practice/Phone

Drugs/Instructions/Signature

SR	SB	ST	SA/B	A FIB	A FL	PAT	SVT	JR	1°	2° A	2° B	3°	VE	R/T	B/T	VT GP	VT PP	VT UN	VF	PVF	IV	AIV	DH	AS	EMD	PM	ISC
A	B	C	D	E	F	G	H	I	J	K	L	M	N	O	P	Q	R	S	T	U	V	W	X	Y	Z	1	2

✓ ON ARRIVAL
X SUBSEQUENT
0 AT HOSPITAL

MANAGEMENT AND REASSESSMENT

Time	Action/Fluid/Drug	Dose	Route	Treatment Effect - Reassessment	L Drug	M Proc.	Officer

FINAL ASSESSMENT	RESPONSE		HANDOVER To: Dr. / RN / Amb.	
	Improved ☐			
	Unchanged ☐		Signature of Ambulance Officer(s)	
	Deteriorated ☐			For Review By ☐

OUTCOME   DOA ☐   Died at Scene ☐   Died en Route ☐   Alive at E/Dept. ☐   Checked by S.O. ☐

2

ABBREVIATIONS

Many words and terms can be abbreviated or represented by a few letters to shorten long descriptions. However, the abbreviations used must be common to medical personnel and not a personal short-cut. Common abbreviations used are shown in the box.

Medical abbreviations for patient care records

Abdo	— abdomen
AMI	— acute myocardial infarction
C	— cervical spine
Ca	— cancer
CCF	— congestive cardiac failure
COAD	— chronic obstructive airways disease
CT	— computerised tomography
CVA	— cerebrovascular accident
DOA	— dead on arrival
#	— fracture
Hx	— history
L	— lumbar spine
Ⓛ	— left
Lac	— laceration
LOC	— loss of consciousness
NOF	— neck of femur
♂	— male
♀	— female
OD	— overdose
OE	— on examination
PR	— per rectum
PV	— per vagina
Ⓡ	— right
Rx	— treatment
SOB	— short of breath
T	— thoracic spine

CASE HISTORY

It is a warm evening and so far the shift has been quiet. You and your crewmate are on station and have just heated a frozen pizza in the microwave. As you sit down to consume your tasty snack, tastebuds tingling, the telephone rings and the controller gives you the following case:

> *I have a motor vehicle crash at the corner of Graham Drive and Wingate Road, Robertsville. Motorcycle and car. Emergency response on case 176, time despatched 2141 hours.*

As a result of the collision, fuel from the motorcycle has ignited, causing a fire hazard. You arrive at the scene 9 minutes after the despatch time, to find a fire brigade unit in attendance and the motorcycle rider lying on the edge of the footpath, several metres from his smouldering motorcycle. A police officer has removed the rider's helmet, covered him with a blanket and is observing him. The occupants of the car are not injured.

1. **What pattern of injury might you expect from the initial information given to you by the controller, as you proceed to the scene?**

2. **On arrival at the scene, what danger(s) may be present and need to be controlled?**

Your primary survey indicates that the rider, a male in his early 20s, is not responding to command, but has a clear airway, is breathing and has a pulse. There is no evidence of significant external bleeding. However, you note that his left leg is severely angulated above the knee.

3. **What judgement do you make from this primary survey and what is your next step?**

You commence a vital signs survey and the physiological assessment reveals:

pulse—120 weak
respirations—30 shallow, non-retractive
blood pressure—85 systolic
capillary refill—2 seconds
eye opening to pain stimulus
verbal response—incomprehensible
motor response—purposeful to pain

4. **What judgement do you make from this part of the vital signs survey and what criteria did you use to make the judgement?**

5. **Is the patient time critical?**

6. **Is the pattern of injury identified of major significance?**

7. **Is the potential injury as judged from the mechanism of injury of major significance?**

8. **Do your observations from the pattern of injury and the potential injury confirm that the patient is time critical?**

9. What management plan might you use, including what further observations you would take?

10. What would you include in your handover at the hospital?

Turn to page 299 to check your answers.

CHAPTER 3
Homeostasis

Clinical problem management in the pre-hospital care environment is aimed at the restoration of homeostasis—the balance within the body. This chapter provides an overview of the mechanisms of balance with an emphasis towards those which relate more directly to pre-hospital intervention.

The accepted ranges of normal physiological values provide a basis for understanding the physiological being before considering clinical problem areas.

Topics covered

Definition of homeostasis
Homeostatic mechanisms
Acid-base balance
Normal physiological values

The human body is a complex organism, comprising many structures which work together. The relationships between the various parts and their functions enables the organism to respond and adapt to changes in the external environment.

Aim

To develop an understanding of the maintenance of balance within the human body

Learning plan

1. Read the text information
2. Conduct the investigative tasks as indicated in the text

DEFINITION OF HOMEOSTASIS

Homeostasis can be defined as 'a tendency to stability in the normal physiological states of the organism' (Dorland's Medical Dictionary). That is to say that the body maintains a balance of its internal environment to function efficiently and in a coordinated manner. Such a balance exists when the internal environment:

- has the correct concentrations of gases, nutrients, ions and water
- has the optimum temperature
- has an optimal pressure for the health and function of cells.

Any disturbance to this balance will result in ill health and if not restored, may cause death.

Emergency care is about the restoration (where possible) of homeostasis, or at the very least, preventing further deterioration of this 'internal environment'. We are exposed to a wide variety of stimuli every day, most of which have some influence on our homeostatic balance. But we are rarely aware of the effects of these stimuli, because of the inherent abilities of our body to compensate, overcome or adapt to the stresses, restoring the balance once more. The inherent abilities of the body are known as homeostatic mechanisms, which are a combination of a variety of body systems and their functions, working in a coordinated manner under the control of the brain.

HOMEOSTATIC MECHANISMS

Consider the athletes competing in Olympic games, especially in high altitude places like Mexico City, or those people who must conquer high mountains where the oxygen level in the atmosphere is reduced. Yet our atheletes and the mountaineers adapt to the new altitude and function normally and efficiently once acclimatised. This process is a homeostatic mechanism—the adaptive mechanism to oxygen lack. Oxygen utilization and carbon dioxide production is greatest when the cells are very active. Maintaining oxygen levels and reducing carbon dioxide to acceptable levels in the extracellular fluid means that respiratory function must increase.

The cardiovascular system (the heart and blood vessels) keeps a constant movement of fresh fluid to all parts of the body. During the stress of physical activity, muscles need more nutrients more rapidly. An increase in the heart rate and the calibre of the arterioles supplying the skeletal muscle areas therefore compensates for the increased demands on the body.

During periods of high physical activity, the body generates heat. The normal internal environment temperature is within a range (37° Celsius, plus or minus 2°). Yet the external environment temperature may vary from $45^\circ C$ to sub-zero levels in the populated regions of our planet. The body's temperature regulatory mechanisms conserve heat in the cold environment and shed heat when the world around is hot. Think about your body's response when you are cold. Shivering (the muscle tremors you experience) generates heat through muscle activity, therefore assisting in the restoration of heat lost to the environment.

Another example of a homeostatic mechanism is nutrient regulation. Along with adequate oxygen, cells need fuel in order to function. The digestive and related accessory organs break down foods into usable components. Some organs, e.g., the liver, store nutrients for later use by body cells, thereby providing a mechanism to restore the balance as required from time to time. The liver stores glucose, the essential cell fuel. The autonomic nervous system maintains a constant surveillance of levels and demands (feedback systems) so that as blood sugar levels vary, stored glucose is released from the liver to restore the balance.

And so it goes with all functions in the body being monitored and actions modified to keep a constant state of physiological balance—*homeostasis*.

3

ACID-BASE BALANCE

The fluids of the body must maintain a fairly constant balance of acids and bases (alkalis). In solutions, such as those found in body cells or in extracellular fluids, acids and bases dissociate into positive and negative particles. If the number of positive particles (hydrogen) is greater, then the solution is acidic. Conversely, if the number of negative particles (hydroxide) is greater, the solution is basic (or alkaline).

Reactions which occur in living systems (biochemical reactions) are extremely sensitive to small changes in the acidity or alkalinity of their environment. Positive and negative particles are involved in practically all biochemical processes and the functions of cells are modified significantly by any departure from the narrow limits of normal particle concentrations. For this reason, the acids and bases which are constantly formed in the body must be kept in balance.

The term *pH* is used to describe the degree of acidity or alkalinity (basicity) of a solution. This is measured on a scale (pH scale), which ranges from 0 to 14 (Fig. 3.1 on page 48). The scale measures the concentration of hydrogen particles in solution. A pH reading of 7 indicates that there are equal numbers of hydrogen and hydroxide particles. For example, water contains 1 hydrogen particle (H^+) and 1 hydroxide particle (OH^-), which exists as H_2O.

Blood pH is normally 7.3-7.4 and it is therefore a fluid containing slightly fewer hydrogen particles, and thus is slightly alkaline. On the other hand, gastric juices, which break down foods into usable substances, have a normal pH of 1.2-3.0. This means that the hydrogen particle concentration is very high and therefore the solution is acidic.

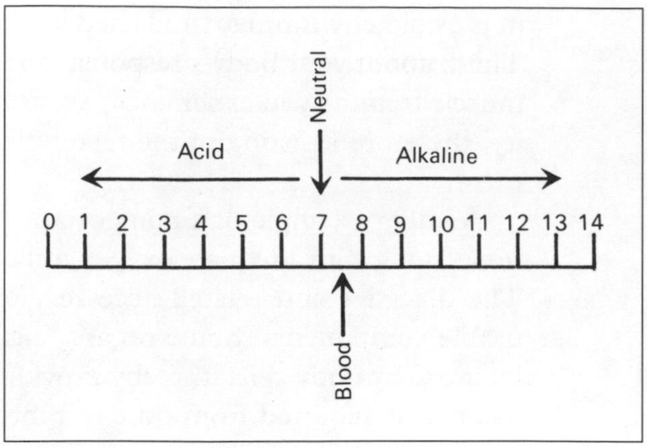

Fig. 3.1 The pH scale. (Reproduced with permission from Wilson K J W 1990 Ross & Wilson: Anatomy and physiology in health and illness, 7th edition. Churchill Livingstone, Edinburgh)

Although the pH of the body fluids may differ, the normal limits for the various fluids are generally quite specific and narrow. Even though strong acids and bases are continually taken into the body, the pH levels of these body fluids remain relatively constant.

The homeostatic mechanisms which maintain pH values in the body are called *buffer systems*. The essential function of a buffer system is to react with strong acids or bases in the body and replace them with weak acids or bases, which alter the pH only slightly. The chemicals which replace strong acids or bases for weak ones are called buffers and are found in the body fluids.

The most important of these buffer systems, which are found in the extracellular fluid, is the *carbonic acid—bicarbonate buffer system*. This consists of a pair of compounds, one a weak acid (carbonic acid H_2CO_3) and the other a weak base (sodium bicarbonate $NaHCO_3$). If the body's pH is threatened by the presence of a strong acid, the weak base of the pair goes into operation. Conversely, if the pH is threatened by the presence of a strong base, the weak acid comes into play.

NORMAL PHYSIOLOGICAL VALUES

When homeostasis is interrupted, the body systems respond to restore the balance. This means that there is a constant state of adjustment which is evidenced by physiological changes in the values of vital functions. Therefore exact values for each of the vital functions is impossible to specify. However, a range of acceptable values for normal functions is used as a guide to determine when normal homeostatic mechanisms are no longer compensating for stresses and insults.

The assessment of physiological status, then, can be made by comparing the recorded values of a patient against the known, accepted normal values.

Normal physiological values (adult)

Respiratory rate	=	12-16 per minute
Pulse rate	=	60-80 per minute
Blood pressure	=	100-160 mmHg

Further physiological data and accepted normal values for paediatric classifications are discussed in the following clinical chapters.

INVESTIGATIVE TASKS

1. Rest for about 5 minutes and have your pulse, breathing and blood pressure recorded. Note also your skin temperature
2. Go for a brisk run or climb several flights of stairs for about 5 minutes
3. Stop and have your pulse, breathing and blood pressure recorded again. Note the changes, including skin temperature
4. Rest again for about 5 minutes and have your pulse, breathing and blood pressure recorded again. Note the changes
5. What do you conclude from this information?

3

CHAPTER 4
Of behaviour

Behavioural disturbance, like homeostatic imbalance, often requires pre-hospital intervention. This chapter describes behavioural variances and the approach to patients, especially the combative patient.

Topics covered

Influences on behaviour
Deviation from normal
Approach to the disturbed patient
The suicidal patient

4

Aim

To develop an understanding of human behaviour and an approach to dealing with abnormal behaviour

Learning plan

1. **Read the text information**
2. **Observe the behaviour patterns of people around you**

Humans are complex beings with equally complex behaviour patterns. Codes of behaviour vary from social group to social group and between cultures and sub-cultures. The definition of 'normal' behaviour then is dependent upon a wide range of variables, circumstances and social conditions relating to the time at which the behaviour is observed. Judgements about 'abnormal' behaviour then must take into account these issues.

INFLUENCES ON BEHAVIOUR

Society consists of a broad cultural mix with different customs and conventions. For example, a Muslim considers it quite normal (through religious teachings) not to eat or even touch pork, because it is 'unclean' and could become very distressed at the thought of doing so.

However, a Christian behaving in this manner might be considered to be 'abnormal'.

Behaviour varies according to our life experience, family patterns and personalities. A strict religious upbringing tends to develop respect for authority, whereas a very casual, non-authoritarian family upbringing may give rise to quite different behaviour. However, this does not imply that the variations are abnormal, merely different. Behaviour which might be defined as 'abnormal' can be explored more closely through three factors, which should be considered together:

1. The circumstances in which the behaviour occurs. For example, it is accepted that an individual will exhibit sadness and even depression at the loss of a close friend or relative. On the other hand, it might be abnormal if the person displayed these behaviours for no apparent reason.

2. The duration of behavioural patterns, such as anger. Following an argument with another individual, anger may not be unusual and might even be justifiable. But this anger is usually short-lived and the event is over in a reasonable time. If, however, the anger was sustained for a long period—well beyond what seems reasonable—then the behaviour might be considered abnormal.

3. The intensity of the behaviour might also be considered abnormal if it is disproportionate to the event. Using the example of anger, a prolonged or even violent rage over a minor argument might not be considered to be a normal behavioural response.

DEVIATION FROM NORMAL

If we consider human behaviour to be within a continuum and that all normal people exhibit a range of behaviour then by identifying the deviations from 'normal' (if sustained and forming the dominant behaviour) we have the basis for classifying mental illness.

The continuum cannot be defined as three clear zones. We may regularly experience anxiety and impulsiveness, but does this mean that we are neurotic? However, if these were the dominant features of our behaviour, then a neurotic classification could be applied.

Normal	Mild	Moderate	Severe
Realistic self image	Anxiety		Personality
Realistic perceptions	Difficulty with concepts		disorganisation
Competence	Difficulty in problem		Delusions
Self acceptance	solving		Hallucinations
Confidence	Self preoccupation		Loss of touch with
Self reliance	Excessive dependency		reality
	needs		
	Impulsive		
NORMAL BEHAVIOUR	NEUROSIS		PSYCHOSIS

Fig. 4.1 The range of behaviour deviations from normal. Neurosis is a disorder of emotion. Psychosis is a disorder of the mind itself.

APPROACH TO THE DISTURBED PATIENT

Dealing with the behaviourally disturbed person requires a patient, concerned approach. Take time to listen to the patient and to learn what it is that is bothering them. The patient with emotional disturbance is usually aware of the problem and the need for help.

The most effective manner in dealing with the aggressive patient is to identify early, the aggression and prevent the patient from becoming combative. Is the patient:

- Agitated, elated or restless
- Demanding constant attention from those around
- Talking loudly or boisterously
- Teasing and baiting others with sarcasm
- Using abusive or vulgar language
- Exhibiting a limited span of attention?

Do not try to control or suppress the behaviour. This may precipitate a combative response. Give the patient room to express feelings:

- Listen, but do not respond to provocative comments or foul language
- Try not to show disapproval to the patient's words or actions
- Do not use complex explanations and ideas; rather, speak in short simple sentences
- Try to remain calm and relaxed. Do not exhibit defensive or aggressive behaviour
- Be careful using gestures or non-verbal signals. Positive signals, such as smiling and nodding may communicate the reverse of that which you intend (e.g., a smile may be misinterpreted by the agitated patient to mean that you are laughing at the patient)
- Make firm decisions.

These steps may assist in keeping you in control of the situation. If the patient becomes combative, despite your best efforts, the patient is now in control and quick action may be necessary:

- Call for assistance, but ensure that others do not intrude unless it becomes necessary. However, they should be aware of what you are doing at all times
- Personal protection is a prime consideration. Ensure that an escape route is available and that you are well clear of any potential weapons. Under no circumstances should you turn your back to the patient
- Do not sound authoritarian and avoid making threats or raising your voice
- Check your progress in resolving the situation by moving closer to the patient and watching for a reaction. If the patient becomes more combative, back away immediately to avoid invading the patient's personal space
- Listen and respond to the patient with empathy, but do not make false promises.

If these steps are unsuccessful, intervention by the police may be the only alternative.

The mental health legislation enables a medical practitioner to commit a behaviourally disturbed patient to a psychiatric centre for further investigation and care. This process requires the provision of correct documentation to be forwarded with the patient. It is essential that these documents are complete and are signed by the doctor before the patient is transported. The provisions of the mental health legislation vary from country to country, and from State to State in Australia, and should be known by the ambulance officer to ensure that all legal requirements are met.

Physical restraint should be used only as a last resort and only then if the patient has been certified by a medical practitioner. Emergency sedation should only be used under medical supervision and is normally not the province of the ambulance officer.

THE SUICIDAL PATIENT

Suicide and attempted suicide are increasing in frequency in most Western countries. This is also true of Australia, and of major concern is the fact that the majority of the victims are young people, in the age range of 15 to 30 years.

The suicidal patient often has feelings of low esteem and worthlessness, unable to deal with the issues of life. Alcoholism and depression, often associated with family separation (death of a loved-one or divorce), are frequently the source of high risk of suicide.

Attempted suicide requires firstly attending to medical treatment. Bleeding must be controlled. Respiratory care is the first priority in drug overdose.

The conscious patient requires empathy. Talk with the patient about the attempt and the problems which might have lead to the situation. Avoid making judgements or suggestions that the action was ill-founded, as this may cause further depression and withdrawal. Reassure the patient and transport quietly to the emergency department and handover to the attending medical officer all relevant information. If drug overdose is attempted, bring to the emergency department all containers and medications which might help in identifying the nature of the poison.

Suicide threats must always be taken seriously and managed with empathy and in a non-judgemental manner.

FURTHER READING

Greenberg M, Szmukler G, Tantam D 1986 Making sense of psychiatric cases. Oxford University Press, Oxford

Goodwin D W, Guze S B 1989 Psychiatric diagnosis. Oxford University Press, Oxford

SECTION 2
Clinical problems

This section covers the main clinical areas in pre-hospital care. Anatomy and physiology are dealt with only in relation to the specific problems discussed. For further information you should refer to more comprehensive texts on the structure and functions of the human body.

CHAPTER 5
Of breathing status

Airway obstruction is the most commonly encountered problem in the respiratory aspect of homeostasis, due to both trauma and disease. Chapter 2 introduced life support intervention for the management of upper airway problems, so the focus in this chapter is on the lower airway.

Trauma, along with disease processes which result in poor or inadequate respiratory status, are discussed. Assessing respiratory status against the normal values provides the basis for judgement. Oxygen therapy and IPPV complete the practical direction of the chapter.

Topics covered

The airway at a glance
Obstruction of the airway
Respiratory function at a glance
Mechanism damage
Gases and gas exchange
The problem of hypoxia
Assessing respiratory status
Oxygen therapy
A few words on suction
The clinical problem of asthma
Chronic obstructive airways disease
The problem of pulmonary oedema

Aim

To develop an understanding of the respiratory pathways and skills in managing airway problems

Learning plan

1. **Read each segment of the text information**
2. **Supplement reading in anatomy and physiology with a more comprehensive text**
3. **Check your understanding using the knowledge checks**
4. **Practise the skills using the skills guides as a reference to check your competence**

The supply of oxygen and the removal of carbon dioxide is a crucial element in the maintenance of homeostasis. Without oxygen, cellular metabolism is non-existent. The movement of air between the atmosphere and the lungs is dependent upon the integrity of the airway.

THE AIRWAY AT A GLANCE

When air is inspired, it is conducted to the lungs through a series of structures known as the airway. Therefore the prime function of the airway is to ensure an air supply line for the body.

THE UPPER AIRWAY

The upper airway consists of the nose and the pharynx (Fig. 5.1). The nose consists of two hollow cavities, separated by a partition (the septum). Each of these cavities is divided into 3 passages by bony projections (turbinates), from the lateral walls of the two cavities.

A ciliated mucous membrane lines the nose (and indeed the remainder of the airway as far as the smaller bronchioles). Air entering through the nose is filtered, warmed and humidified before reaching the lungs.

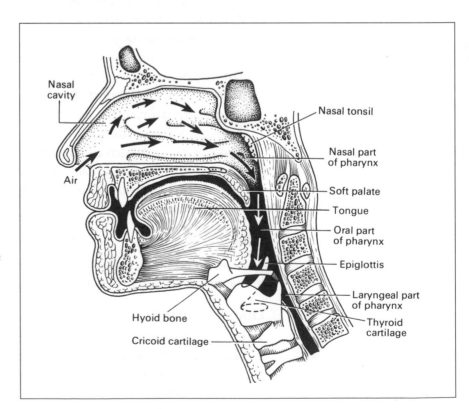

Fig. 5.1 Cross-section of the upper airway with arrows showing the movement of air from the nose to the larynx. (Reproduced with permission from Wilson K J W 1990 Ross & Wilson: Anatomy and physiology in health and illness, 7th edition. Churchill Livingstone, Edinburgh)

The pharynx. This is the tube-like structure extending from the base of the skull to the commencement of the larynx and lies anterior to the cervical spine. This muscular structure, lined with mucous membrane, has three anatomical divisions:

- The nasopharynx, posterior to the nasal cavities and above the soft palate
- The oropharynx, bordered by the soft palate above and to the level of the hyoid bone below
- The laryngopharynx, continuous with the oropharynx and the common site for foreign body obstruction.

The pharynx is the common passageway for both food and air. To ensure that food and air enter the appropriate tubes, a small leaf shaped projection attached to the thyroid cartilage, the *epiglottis*, protects the airway during swallowing.

Inspection of the upper airway with a laryngoscope or lighted spatula will show the significant landmarks of the oropharynx (Fig. 5.2). Progressing over the tongue and viewing laterally, behind the pillars of the fauces, we can see:

- The palatine tonsils
- The end segment of the soft palate, the uvula, is clearly seen midline.

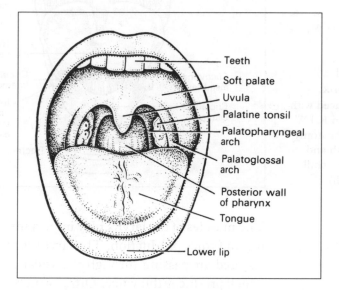

Fig. 5.2 Anatomical landmarks of the oropharynx. (Reproduced with permission from Wilson K J W 1990 Ross & Wilson: Anatomy and physiology in health and illness, 7th edition. Churchill Livingstone, Edinburgh)

Advancing the tip of the laryngoscope over the base of the tongue will bring into view the epiglottis. Placing the tip of the blade into the vallecula groove and with careful jaw thrust, the *vocal cords* of the larynx can be seen.

Managing upper airway obstruction was dealt with in Chapter 2.

THE LOWER AIRWAY

The lower airway consists of a series of muscular tubes, some ringed with cartilage, whose purpose is to conduct air to and from the terminal sacs (alveoli) in the lungs.

The larynx. Also known as the voice box, this lies at the root of the tongue and is guarded by the epiglottis (Fig. 5.3). The larynx consists largely of cartilages, the two largest being:

- Thyroid cartilage, (or Adam's apple) is the larger and creates the characteristic triangular shape anteriorly
- Cricoid cartilage, which lies inferior to the thyroid cartilage with its shape resembling a signet ring.

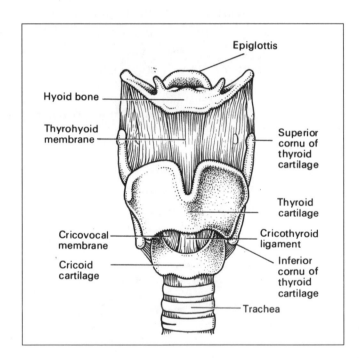

Fig. 5.3 Anatomical structures of the larynx. Front view. (Reproduced with permission from Wilson K J W 1990 Ross & Wilson: Anatomy and physiology in health and illness, 7th edition. Churchill Livingstone, Edinburgh)

The muscles of the larynx play important roles in ventilation, swallowing and voice production. The larynx is the organ of voice production. Expired air passing through the vocal cords causes them to vibrate, which produces the voice. Other structures such as the nose, mouth, pharynx and the bony sinuses of the skull act as sounding boards which help determine voice quality.

The trachea. Also known as the windpipe, this is a tube ringed by cartilage, approximately 11cm in length and with a diameter of about 2.5 cm. It extends from the larynx to the level of the second costal cartilage. The trachea ensures an open airway to the lungs and divides at its inferior end into two main bronchi (Fig. 5.4). The right main bronchus is slightly larger and more vertical than the left main bronchus. Hence, aspirated foreign bodies more frequently lodge in the right main bronchus. The structure of the bronchi is similar to the trachea, and they are lined with ciliated mucosa.

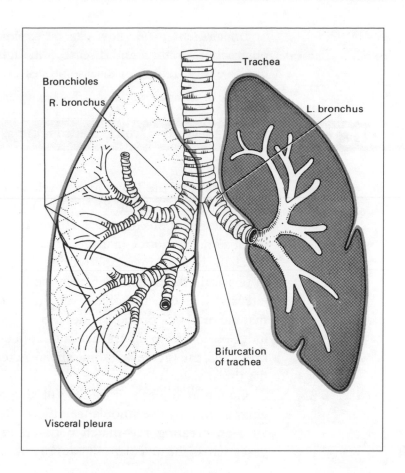

Fig. 5.4 The bronchial tree and lungs. (Reproduced with permission from Wilson K J W 1990 Ross & Wilson: Anatomy and physiology in health and illness, 7th edition. Churchill Livingstone, Edinburgh)

5

The small bronchi and bronchioles. Each main bronchus divides into smaller branches immediately after entering the lungs. The smaller bronchi continue to branch, forming the small, smooth muscled tubes called bronchioles. The small bronchi and bronchioles function in the same manner as the trachea and main bronchi distributing inspired air to the lungs.

The alveoli. The bronchioles sub-divide into microscopic branches, alveolar ducts and terminate as alveolar sacs. The sac consists of many alveoli and can be likened to a bunch of grapes. The alveoli are enveloped by networks of capillaries and it is here that the vital function of gas exchange takes place (Fig. 5.5).

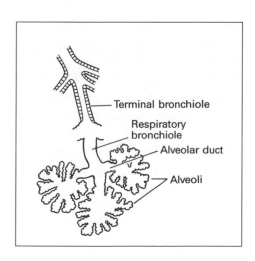

Fig. 5.5 Diagram of the bronchioles and alveoli. (Reproduced with permission from Wilson K J W 1990 Ross & Wilson: Anatomy and physiology in health and illness, 7th edition. Churchill Livingstone, Edinburgh)

Impairment to air flow can be explored under the headings of obstruction, trauma and disease, although essentially, obstruction is due to either trauma or disease processes.

OBSTRUCTION OF THE AIRWAY

Obstruction of the lower airway relates more commonly to disease process than to foreign body obstruction, although inhaled or impacted obstructions do occur. However, objects below the level of the vocal cords cannot be managed in the pre-hospital environment with much success and invariably require surgical intervention. In the event of physical obstruction by foreign body, attempts to forcefully ventilate and dislodge the object should be made following the use of manual methods previously described. Forceful ventilation may dislodge objects from the trachea and reduce the obstruction to the right bronchus, thus achieving some airway patency to eliminate immediate life threat risk.

Common disease processes (of the obstructive kind) regularly encountered by the ambulance officer affect the smaller airways and air-sacs, creating mis-match between ventilation and diffusion of gases across the alveolar (air-sac) membrane.

FOREIGN OBJECTS

Inhalation of foreign objects which lodge in the larynx or indeed lower in the respiratory pathway poses varying degrees of emergency in the pre-hospital care setting. An object lodged in the narrow confines of the larynx may result in obstruction due to stimulation of the muscles of the larynx to contract in spasm. Manual clearing methods (back blows or abdominal thrusts) may dislodge some foreign objects, but those below the vocal cords are not likely to be successfully removed by manual means at our disposal in the field. Forceful ventilation may dislodge the object and move the obstruction into the right bronchus, thus achieving an air pathway to the left lung fields adequate to sustain respiratory function until surgical removal by bronchoscopy can be performed in the hospital.

Following successful removal of a foreign object from the airway, transport to the emergency department is important to ensure that no further respiratory impairment exists. Foreign objects impacted in the tissues of the airway do cause tissue damage and swelling, which may result in further airway problems.

TRAUMA

Trauma to the lower airway more commonly effects the larynx. Blunt trauma to the neck may result in crush injury to the cartilaginous segments, narrowing the airway and causing tissue oedema or possibly laryngeal spasm. Penetrating injuries may also result in interruption of the air pathway due to bleeding and oedema of damaged tissues. Aspiration of fluids and the inhalation of fumes and hot gases will also irritate the mucosa, resulting in oedema and hence obstruction. Fluids and petroleum products (e.g., kerosine) may also cause obstruction to the diffusion of gases across the respiratory membrane in addition to the irritation of mucosa.

DISEASE

Disease processes are a common cause of airway impairment. Of significance is asthma. Obstruction occurs as a result of all three elements of the pathology—bronchospasm, mucosal oedema and mucous plugging of the smaller, muscular walled bronchioles. The use of potent bronchodilators such as salbutamol early in the asthma episode may relieve the obstructive effects in the short term, but hospital management of the remaining pathology is essential. (See asthma, page 83.) Bronchitis and tracheitis, while rarely causing complete obstruction, may result in restriction of the air pathway to the extent of causing severe dyspnoea. Pneumonia, while a disease process affecting lung tissue rather than the airway, may produce thick sputum which plugs the smaller bronchioles, adding an obstructive element to the disease. Emphysema is classified as a chronic obstructive airways disease, but the pathology relates to the destruction of alveoli, reducing the diffusion surface area of the lungs. The effect is more a mismatch between ventilation and diffusion, rather than a failure of the airway to deliver inspired air to the alveoli. (See emphysema, page 88.)

Tumours can develop in most tissues. Growths forming in the lumen of the air pathways cause progressive narrowing and often total obstruction. These are normally 'pre-diagnosed' and the ambulance officer's contact with such patients is usually in the transportation to hospital for admission or outpatient treatment. In-transit care may require oxygen therapy.

5

RESPIRATORY FUNCTION AT A GLANCE

THE LUNGS

The lungs are the cone-shaped organs of respiration, occupying the pleural cavities of the thorax. Their position in relation to the heart and the major blood vessels is shown in Figure 5.6. They extend from the diaphragm inferiorly to just beyond the clavicular line superiorly and lie against the rib cage anteriorly and posteriorly. Because of this extension beyond the clavicular line, penetrating injuries to the shoulder may involve a lung injury (pneumothorax). Each lung is divided into lobes—the left lung comprises two lobes and the right, three lobes. The outer surface of the lungs is covered by the pleural membrane which has two layers:

- the visceral pleura, adhering to the outer surface of the lung
- the parietal pleura, adhering to the inner surface of the thoracic wall and diaphragm.

The two layers of the pleural membrane are in close proximity to each other and separated only by a potential space. The cohesion between the layers of the pleura is important for the expansion and recoil of the lungs as the chest wall and diaphragm move. Loss of this cohesion will result in partial or complete collapse of the lung.

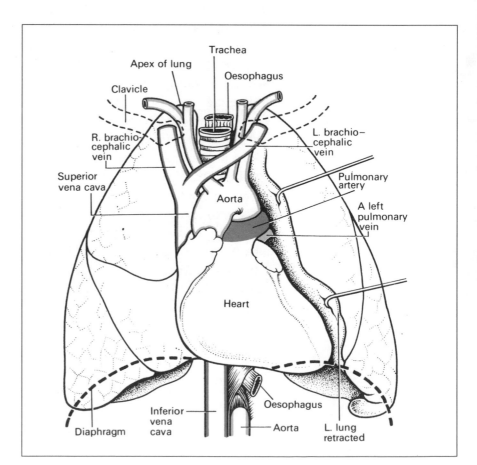

Fig. 5.6 The relationship of the lungs to the other structures of the thorax. Note the position of the clavicle. (Reproduced with permission from Wilson K J W 1990 Ross & Wilson: Anatomy and physiology in health and illness, 7th edition. Churchill Livingstone, Edinburgh)

MECHANISM OF BREATHING

Normal (quiet) inspiration is caused by contraction of the diaphragm, which increases the superior/inferior diameter of the thorax, and contraction of the external intercostal muscles, which increases the anterior/posterior and transverse diameter of the thorax. This movement results in a decrease in interthoracic pressure. The cohesion of the pleura ensures lung expansion, which decreases alveolar pressure. A pressure gradient is created between the atmosphere and the alveoli. Air moves from a high pressure to a low pressure, hence air enters the alveoli—the inspiratory phase.

The mechanism of normal expiration is the reverse process. Inspirational muscles relax, decreasing the size of the thorax, resulting in recoil of lung tissue, which increases interthoracic pressure. The decrease in lung size raises alveolar pressure and a pressure gradient is thus created from alveoli to the atmosphere—hence the expiratory phase.

After each expiratory phase, there is a pause of about 3 seconds duration before the next inspiration occurs. This is the respiratory pause.

MECHANISM DAMAGE

5

RIB FRACTURE

One of the most common injuries to the chest wall is rib fracture. Loss of the continuity of the rib cage reduces inspiratory efficiency, which results in decreased lung inflation. If the volume of air entering the lung fields is less, the oxygen diffusion across the respiratory membrane is reduced, thus less oxygen is available to the tissues (hypoxia).

Rib fractures may be simple, without serious damage to underlying or overlying tissues. Pain is the most significant feature because it prevents the patient from taking adequate inspirations. Tenderness at the site of injury is also increased on breathing and coughing.

Treatment

The aim of treatment is to improve oxygenation by supplementing inspired air with oxygen and encouraging the patient to take deep breaths. The administration of pain relief and oxygen, in addition to a comfortable posture which affords maximum ventilation (semi-recumbent, inclined to the injured side), is the first order management approach. There is little to be gained by bandaging the chest to support the rib fracture and in fact this action may reduce the patient's capacity to breathe effectively.

FLAIL CHEST

A flail chest develops when there are several ribs or the sternum fractured in more than one place. The unsupported chest wall segment moves 'paradoxically'. On inspiration, as the chest expands, the segment sinks inward, impairing the ability to draw in air. On exhalation, the segment may bulge outwards, thus impairing the ability to exhale.

In severe cases, air may shift uselessly from side to side in the bronchial tree, further reducing lung inflation. A pneumothorax is frequently associated with a flail chest and examination of respiratory function should always include a check for such lung collapse.

Treatment

Treatment, in addition to the management of the airway and oxygenation, requires stabilisation of the flail segment. This is best achieved by bandaging a bulky pad over the flail area firmly, minimising paradoxical movement and providing some restoration of stability to the chest wall. The severe disruption to respiratory function and the likelihood of pneumothorax with this injury make it a 'time critical' event, requiring urgent treatment and transport to the emergency department.

PNEUMOTHORAX

Complicated rib fractures may involve laceration to the chest wall, pleura and lungs. Penetration of the chest wall, and laceration or tearing of the lung by a penetrating object or rib fragment, may produce a condition where air enters the normally 'potential' space of the pleura, causing the pleura to separate. Air in the thoracic cavity (pneumothorax) causes the lung on the affected side to progressively collapse inwards. Mediastinal shift gradually compresses the opposite lung and impairs its ventilation. Haemothorax (an accumulation of blood in the pleural cavity) frequently accompanies pneumothorax and is seen in both open and closed chest injury.

Pneumothorax can also occur spontaneously. A congenitally weak area of the lung surface may rupture, resulting in a sudden sharp chest pain and respiratory difficulty.

Treatment

The first order management of pneumothorax is maintenance of adequate oxygenation by posture and supplemented oxygen. If the patient is in severe respiratory distress with a tachycardia (rapid pulse) and is hypotensive (low blood pressure), decompression of the chest is urgent. Respiratory support and rapid transport to the emergency department is required.

TENSION PNEUMOTHORAX

If lung tissue or the chest wall is penetrated, forming a 'one-way valve' effect, air entering the pleural space during inspiration cannot escape during exhalation. The resulting pressure build up may collapse the lung completely, causing marked mediastinal shift, which compresses the opposite lung. This tension pneumothorax will result in the air pressure within the thoracic cavity continuing to rise and as mediastinal shift increases, the venae cava become kinked and restricted, impairing the venous return to the heart. This effect is evidenced by marked dyspnoea (difficulty in breathing), tachycardia, hypotension and distension of the veins in the neck. Subcutaneous emphysema (air in the subcutaneous tissues) is often present and in severe cases can produce a grotesque appearance with the entire chest as well as the face and neck bloated.

Treatment

Again, this injury is 'time critical' and requires urgent transport to the emergency department for chest decompression. Oxygen therapy at the highest concentration possible is essential to maintain respiratory function.

5

OPEN CHEST WOUNDS

Open chest wounds may result in the air being sucked into the chest cavity during inspiration and forced out through the opening during exhalation. This produces a characteristic 'sucking' noise. As air moves into the chest cavity, it creates a pneumothorax and if there is associated bleeding, a haemothorax.

Treatment

The priority in management is to prevent air entering through the opening. This can be achieved quickly and effectively by covering the opening with an air-occlusive dressing. But, if the dressing is sealed on all four sides, there is a risk of producing a tension pneumothorax. The base of the dressing should be left unsealed so that a one-way valve is created, allowing air to escape during exhalation but preventing entry during inspiration. The patient should be positioned so that the valve dressing is not restricted and oxygen administration is again a vital requirement.

DIAPHRAGM INJURY

Diaphragm injury is commonly due to penetrating wounds to the lower chest and upper abdomen, although bullet wounds in other regions of the trunk may reach the diaphragm, depending on the trajectory of the missile and whether it was deflected by bony structures. Rupture of the diaphragm may result from severe blunt trauma to similar regions of the body.

Treatment

The diaphragm produces the greatest proportion of ventilatory activity and therefore the patient may require assisted ventilation during treatment and transport to maintain effective tidal flow and oxygenation.

GASES AND GAS EXCHANGE

The atmosphere around us has weight and is measured as pressure (atmospheric pressure). The pressure at sea level (i.e., one atmosphere) is 760 mm of mercury (Hg). Air is a mixture of gases:

- oxygen (O_2)   about 21%
- nitrogen (N)   about 78%
- carbon dioxide (CO_2)   about 0.04%
- other gases   about 0.96%

Each gas in the mixture exerts its own pressure depending on its concentration and this is referred to as *partial pressure* (Dalton's law). Of the gases in the air, oxygen is essential for respiration and life support.

If oxygen is 21% of the atmosphere, then the partial pressure of oxygen in the atmosphere (PO_2) is:

$$\frac{21 \times 760}{100} = 159.6 \ (160 \ \text{mmHg})$$

Carbon dioxide is exhaled as a by-product of cellular metabolism. If carbon dioxide is 0.04% of the atmosphere, then the partial pressure of carbon dioxide in the atmosphere (PCO_2) is:

$$\frac{0.04 \times 760}{100} = 0.304 \ (0.3 \ \text{mmHg})$$

During the process of inspiration, the air is modified. The upper respiratory tract, especially the nasal cavity, warms, filters and humidifies the air. Humidification means that the air is saturated with water vapour. Water vapour exerts its own pressure (about 47 mmHg) and therefore the percentages of gases in the alveoli are modified. Further, the 'anatomical dead space'—that part of the airway in which no gas exchange occurs—contains gases which results in intermixing with inspired gases, lowering the percentage of oxygen and elevating that of carbon dioxide. Alveolar oxygen is now approximately 14%, and carbon dioxide is 5.5%. Therefore, the PO_2 in the alveoli is:

$$\frac{14 \times (760 - 47)}{100} = 99.8 \text{ mmHg} (100 \text{ mmHg})$$

and PCO_2 is:

$$\frac{5.5 \times (760 - 47)}{100} = 39.2 \text{ mmHg} (40 \text{ mmHg})$$

Gas exchange between inspired air and the blood is the function jointly carried out by the alveoli and the pulmonary capillaries. They are highly efficient in their task because of the huge surface area of the respiratory membrane. It is estimated to be about 85 m², which is in excess of forty times the surface area of the body, or about the size of a doubles tennis court.

The contact between the very thin-walled alveoli and capillaries makes possible rapid diffusion of gases between alveolar air and the blood. Figure 5.7 illustrates the respiratory membrane and the close proximity between alveolar air and the blood in the pulmonary capillary. Oxygen and carbon dioxide in solution within the blood (blood gases) in turn exert pressures. Venous blood entering the lung capillaries contains oxygen at a partial pressure of about 40 mmHg and carbon dioxide at about 46 mmHg. Therefore, pressure gradients exist between alveolar and blood gases, resulting in exchange across the respiratory membrane.

5

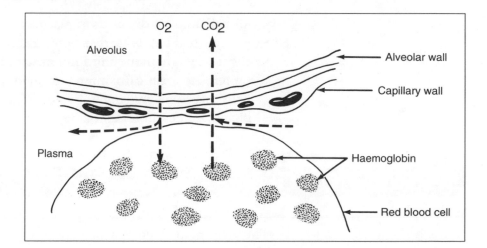

Fig. 5.7 Simplified diagram of the respiratory membrane showing the diffusion of gases between alveolus and red blood cell.

The slow movement of blood through the pulmonary capillary beds allows time for equilibration of gases across the respiratory membrane, i.e., the shift of gases from alveolar air into solution and vice-versa, to a state of approximate balance.

The amount of gas exchange is dependent not only upon the pressure gradients, but also upon:

- the total functional surface area of the respiratory membrane
- alveolar ventilation.

Arterial blood leaving the lung capillaries contains oxygen at a partial pressure of about 100 mmHg and carbon dioxide at about 40 mmHg.

GAS TRANSPORT

Oxygen entering the pulmonary capillaries immediately dissolves in blood plasma. However, most combines chemically with haemo-globin, the principal agent of red blood cells. Haemoglobin affinity to oxygen (1 gram of haemoglobin can unite with 1.34 ml of oxygen) enables large amounts of oxygen to combine to form oxyhaemoglobin. The amount of oxygen in the blood depends essentially on the amount of haemoglobin present. Normally, 100 ml of blood contains approxi-mately 15 grams of haemoglobin. Thus, arterial oxygen contains about 20 ml of oxygen in each 100 ml of blood.

By the time blood leaves the pulmonary capillaries to return to the heart, approximately 97% of the blood's haemoglobin has combined with oxygen (i.e., normal oxygen saturation is close to 100%.). In this combined state, oxygen is transported to the cellular level, where transfer between the cell and the blood occurs.

Carbon dioxide is transported in several ways in the blood. The three most significant forms of transport are:

- a small amount dissolves in plasma
- greater than half is carried as bicarbonate ions in plasma
- slightly less than one-third unites with haemoglobin and other proteins to form carbaminohaemoglobin (not to be confused with carboxyhaemoglobin, which is the combination of haemo-globin with carbon monoxide).

REGULATION OF BREATHING

There are many factors which contribute to the control of breathing. They are considered in three main groups—chemical, nervous and other factors.

Chemical factors

Partial pressure of carbon dioxide (PCO_2)
An increase in arterial blood carbon dioxide stimulates chemoreceptor cells (specialised cells which react to chemical stimulus) in the brain and peripherally (in the carotid bodies and the aorta). Small shifts in

PCO_2 above the normal range of 38-40 mmHg affect the central chemoreceptors in the medulla (in the brainstem). Much larger increases stimulate the peripheral chemoreceptors. Thus, an increased PCO_2 results in an increased breathing rate and increased minute volume (the total air breathed in one minute, i.e., the number of breaths in one minute x amount of air moved per breath). The effect of this increased breathing rate then is the means of compensating for reduced oxygen at the cell level or meeting the cell's increased demands during periods of high activity.

Partial pressure of oxygen (PO₂)

Arterial PO_2 is thought to have little influence on breathing regulation while the level remains within normal limits. However, respiratory centre neurones (nerve cells in the medulla), like other cells in the body, require adequate oxygenation to maintain their function. Thus, if the PO_2 falls, cells become hypoxic and their impulse emission to respiratory muscles reduces. The effect is reduced breathing rate and reduced minute volume. If arterial PO_2 falls below 70 mmHg (but not below the critical level of about 60 mmHg) peripheral chemoreceptors (carotid bodies and aorta) are stimulated and cause reflex stimulation of the respiratory centre. This is the emergency mechanism of respiratory control.

Acid-base balance (pH)

The acid-base balance in the body, acts as a stimulator of peripheral chemoreceptors when arterial blood pH decreases (i.e., an increase in blood acidity), resulting in an increased respiratory rate.

Nervous factors

These factors provide the automatic nature of breathing. The respiratory centre, located in the medulla and pons (in the brainstem), initiates impulses that produce regular inspiratory and expiratory phases and is the major factor in breathing. Impulses from other cerebral areas (e.g., the motor cortex and emotional centres) may modify the rate and alter the depth of breathing.

Other regulatory factors

Temperature, pain receptors and stretch receptors in the rib cage, play a minor role in regulating breathing.

KNOWLEDGE CHECK

The airway

1. What is the prime purpose of the airway?

2. What three functions occur in the upper airway?

3. The pharynx is a common passageway for both food and air. What structure protects the airway during swallowing?

4. The larynx consists largely of cartilage. What are the names of the two largest cartilages?

5. The trachea is approximately 11 cm in length, extending from the larynx to the level of which costal cartilage?

6. What is the structural difference between the bronchi and the bronchioles?

7. In which component of the respiratory tract does the vital function of gas exchange occur?

The lungs

8. What are the superior and inferior margins of the lungs?

9. What is the significance of the superior margin of the lungs when considering penetrating injuries?

10. What is the membrane covering the outer surface of the lungs?

11. What is the significance of this membrane?

12. Describe the processes of normal inspiration and normal expiration.

Gases and gas exchange

13. What are the percentages of oxygen and carbon dioxide in the atmosphere?

14. Describe what is meant by the term 'partial pressure'.

15. Given that atmospheric pressure at sea level is 760 mmHg, calculate the partial pressures for oxygen and carbon dioxide.

16. What is meant by the phrase 'anatomical dead space'?

17. Given that water vapour partial pressure is 47 mmHg, oxygen and carbon dioxide percentage in the alveoli are 14% and 5.5% respectively calculate their partial pressures.

18. Apart from pressure gradients, what two factors influence gas exchange?

Turn to page 300 to check your answers.

THE PROBLEM OF HYPOXIA

Hypoxia is the reduction of oxygen at the tissue level below normal physiological levels, despite an adequate perfusion of blood. In the acutely ill or injured patient, hypoxia can significantly reduce the patient's chance of survival. Hypoxia may be caused by reduced respiration or circulatory deficit.

Reduced respiration. This may have the following origin:

- Nervous (disease or injury to the respiratory centre, spinal cord and spinal nerves)
- Mechanical (disease or injury to the chest wall, muscles, pleura and lungs)
- Obstructive (airway blockage, limiting the flow of air to the alveoli)
- Haemoglobin inadequacy (as in carbon monoxide poisoning or anaemia)
- The inability of tissues to use oxygen (as in cyanide poisoning).

Circulatory deficit. This may originate from the following:

- Reduced cardiac efficiency or output
- Inadequate blood volume (as in blood loss)
- Inadequate tissue blood flow.

Clinically, the patient presents with:

- an increased respiratory rate—breathing may be rapid and shallow (as with rib fracture, the rate compensating for a small tidal volume as a consequence of pain)
- pallor, due to the reduced blood supply to the extremities, as vascular compensation occurs
- cyanosis (the bluish tinge to the extremities) which is a late sign and indicative of extreme hypoxia.

Lack of oxygen, whatever the cause, will eventually cause changes in brain function—anxiety, agitation, confusion, irritability, drowsiness and coma. Tachycardia is due to increased carbon dioxide in the blood.

Treatment

Management of hypoxia requires, firstly, attention to those causes which are of a life threatening nature (e.g., airway obstruction, or major bleeding). High flow oxygen therapy is required initially and may be reduced when there is evidence of good tissue perfusion, identified by a return to the normal 'pink' and warm state and adequate capillary refill (see Chapter 6).

5

ASSESSING RESPIRATORY STATUS

Assessment of respiratory status is a clinical observation, consisting of looking at and listening to the patient. The observations will provide both subjective and objective data, which can be compared with known normal values about respiratory function. The difference between the data and normal values helps then in understanding the severity of respiratory dysfunction and indicates the need and extent of immediate patient care and the efficiency of treatment.

NORMAL RESPIRATORY VALUES

The respiratory cycle consists of the duration of inspiration, expiration and the respiratory pause. This cycle in an adult is approximately 4 seconds.

Respiratory cycle

- Inspiratory phase = 0.75 seconds
- Expiratory phase = 0.25 seconds
- Respiratory pause = 3 seconds
- Respiratory rate = the number of respiratory cycles per minute.

The normal rate is 12-16 per minute.

Normal breathing is rhythmic and is observed by looking and feeling for chest wall/abdomen movement. This rhythmic movement is more easily observed by placing one hand over the patient's lower rib margin and upper abdomen (abdominal movement is usually more evident than chest movement).

Breath sounds are normally quiet.

Skin colour and pulse rate, while specifically a part of assessing perfusion status and discussed in Chapter 6, are signs worth considering during respiratory assessment. Normal colour of the skin is 'pink' and warm to touch. Normal pulse rate is 60–80 beats per minute.

Other functions to note are vital capacity and difficulty with speech.

Normal airway status enables us to exercise vital capacity (i.e., maximum inspiration and maximum expiration). Inability to take a deep breath, hold it and then exhale forcefully may help in identifying respiratory problems involving the airway.

Normal respiratory status enables us to speak clearly and steadily and we are alert. Speech difficulties and an alteration of conscious status should also be considered in assessing respiratory status.

| **TASK** | Respiratory status assessment | 264 |

OXYGEN THERAPY

Oxygen is a colourless, odourless gas. Pure or 100% oxygen is obtained commercially by fractional distillation, in which air is liquefied and the gases other than oxygen (principally nitrogen) are boiled off. Liquid oxygen is then converted under high pressure to a gaseous state and stored in suitably sized cylinders.

Gas flow from an oxygen cylinder is controlled by regulators which reduce the high pressure of the gas in the cylinder—up to 15 000 kilopascals (kPa)—to a safe range of about 414 kPa and control the flow so that oxygen may be delivered to a patient at a rate from 1-15 litres per minute. Regulators attach to the cylinder by means of a yoke, which is designed to engage only the type of cylinder for which it was made, thus preventing errors in gas administration.

All gas cylinders are colour-coded according to their contents. For example, oxygen cylinders are black with a white yoke at the top of the cylinder.

SAFETY PRECAUTIONS

5

Oxygen is the principal gas used in pre-hospital care, and as with all gases in pressure cylinders, care is required in its storage and use.

- Combustible materials (e.g., oil and grease) must not be permitted to come into contact with the cylinder or other fittings
- Smoking is not permitted in any area where oxygen cylinders are in use or on standby
- Cylinders should not be subjected to temperatures above 50°C
- Valves should be closed when the cylinder is not in use, even if the cylinder is empty
- Oxygen cylinders should never be used without a safe and properly fitted regulator valve and the valve should not be modified for use with any other gas
- Cylinders should be secured to prevent them from toppling over. In transit, a proper carrier or rack should be fitted or strapped to the stretcher with the patient

A loose fitting regulator valve can be blown off the cylinder with sufficient force to kill or cause serious injury.

NEVER PLACE ANY PART OF YOUR BODY OVER A CYLINDER VALVE NOR POINT THE VALVE AT A PERSON

OXYGEN ADMINISTRATION

The delivery of oxygen to patients in the emergency setting is a vital part of life support. Early intervention with supplementary oxygen will help to reduce the effects of hypoxia and should be maintained until handover at the emergency department.

The use of oxygen masks (Fig. 5.8) enables high flow rates to be administered. Most acutely ill or injured patients should receive oxygen therapy at a rate of 6-8 litres per minute. As with all forms of treatment, monitoring the effect is vital and the rate may be varied once the patient's perfusion and respiratory status improves to within normal, acceptable limits.

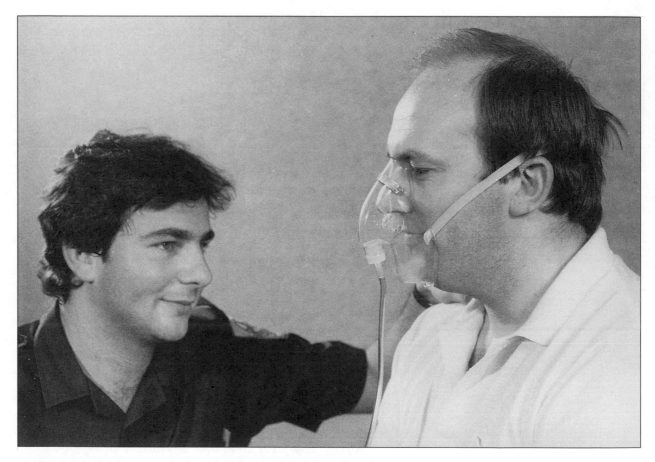

Fig. 5.8 Administering oxygen to a patient using a face mask. The mask should fit snug to the patient's face.

Oxygen delivered by a face mask at 6-8 litres per minute will provide an oxygen concentration of about 40%. An alternative delivery mode is by the use of a nasal cannula (Fig. 5.9). However, the maximum rate tolerated by the patient is 4 litres per minute and this may not be adequate to stabilise the hypoxic problems presented. Flow rates beyond the 4 litres per minute will cause nasal irritation and discomfort.

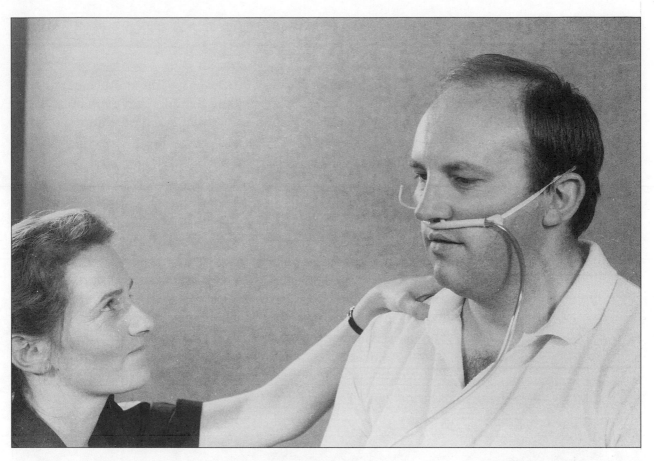

Fig. 5.9 Administering oxygen to a patient using a nasal cannula. The correct position of the prongs in the nose will minimise discomfort.

5

In the pre-hospital care setting, where the duration of care is usually short (in most cases, up to an hour), there is little need for a humidifier. Where long term transport is required, or if so requested by a medical officer transferring a patient, humidified oxygen may be necessary to reduce the drying effects on the mucosa of the patient's mouth and throat.

TASKS		
	1. Assemble an oxygen therapy unit	*Use procedure for own equipment*
	2. Change over oxygen cylinders	*Use procedure for own equipment*
	3. Administer oxygen via a face mask	258
	4. Administer oxygen via a nasal cannula	259

INTERMITTENT POSITIVE PRESSURE VENTILATION (IPPV)

The use of ventilation devices has been part of the ambulance environment for the past 20 years. During this period, many ventilators, some oxygen powered, have been introduced as standard equipment.

Bag-mask devices

Bag-mask devices use atmospheric air (oxygen at 21%) and are self-inflating (Fig. 5.10). However, by attaching an oxygen source to the bag, at a flow rate of 10-12 litres per minute, the oxygen concentration can be elevated to about 40%. Ventilators with a reservoir bag attached are capable of delivering oxygen up to about 90%.

The advantage of using a bag-mask resuscitator as opposed to the expired air resuscitation method is that the rescuer can deliver greater oxygen levels to the patient. The elimination of direct contact with the patient is another significant advantage to the rescuer in that it minimises the risks of transmission of infections. Bag-mask devices are also less tiring for the rescuer.

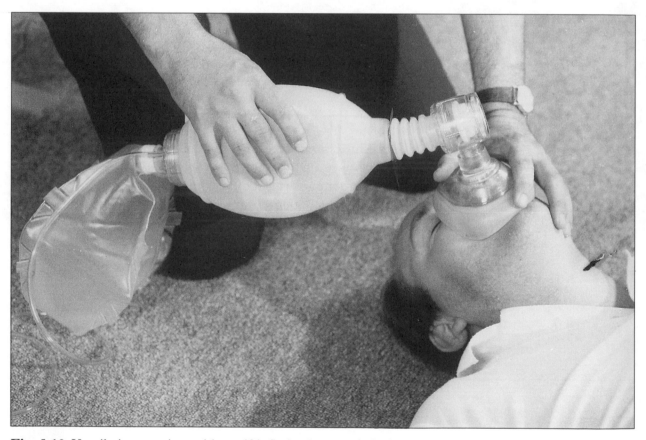

Fig. 5.10 Ventilating a patient with a self-inflating bag-mask device. The reservoir improves oxygen concentration.

Oxygen-powered devices

Oxygen-powered devices generally require large oxygen volume supplies, but have the advantage of being capable of delivering up to 100% oxygen concentration. There are two types of systems in general use: demand valve, and soft bag rebreathing devices.

Demand valve devices (Fig. 5.11) operate by way of a demand valve trigger, which serves two purposes. The rescuer may manually trigger the system to ventilate a non-breathing patient or assist a patient's breathing by direct demand valve function. The demand valve operates when slight negative pressure is created by the patient's inspiratory effort, allows oxygen to be inspired, and on cessation of the negative inspiratory pressure, allows exhaled gases to escape through a non-return valve. The manual triggering method should be used with caution because of the high pressures delivered, which may cause severe gastric distension.

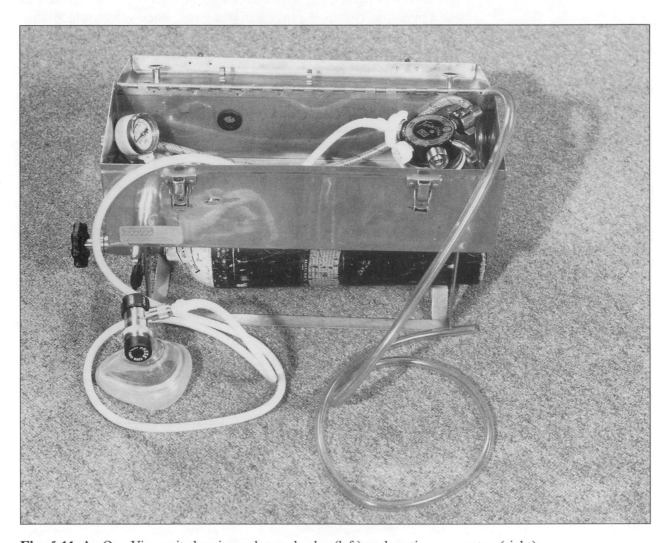

Fig. 5.11 An Oxy-Viva unit showing a demand valve (left) and suction apparatus (right).

Soft bag rebreathing devices utilise the principles of the anaesthetic machines used in the operating theatre (Fig. 5.12). Oxygen pressure is reduced to a safe working pressure (414 kPa) and a closed circuit system recycles exhaled oxygen via a filter, thus conserving oxygen supplies. The flow rate may be varied usually within the range of 0.5-8 litres per minute.

The advantage of this ventilator over demand valve systems, apart from conservation of oxygen, is that soft bag ventilation minimises gastric distension and can be used to monitor respiratory function.

Of particular note is the Komesaroff Oxy-Resuscitator, which provides multiple functions in a single unit. A self-seal outlet at the base of the regulator enables oxygen therapy administration outside the main circuit along with a Venturi suction system. However, the suction unit, being oxygen driven, uses high volumes (about 20 litres per minute) and therefore should be used for short periods only. It is rare to use suction for more than 15 to 20 seconds and as such it is an effective device. A cross valve enables the rescuer to control the circuit and open the system to purge exhaled gases when ventilating victims of toxic gases. A soda lime canister is used in the closed circuit configuration to filter carbon dioxide from expired air, returning oxygen into the circuit.

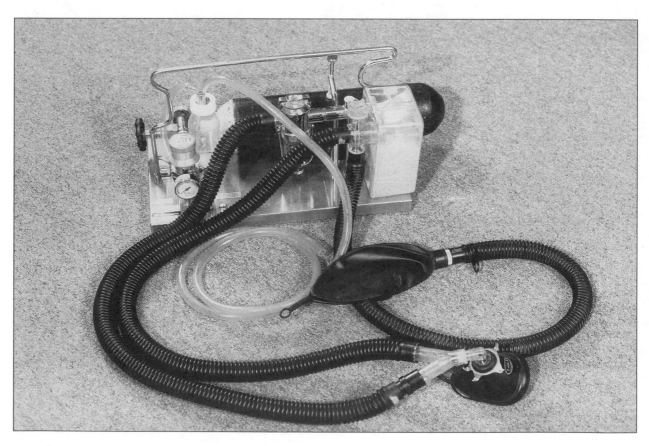

Fig. 5.12 A soft bag rebreathing unit (Oxy-Resuscitator).

Time-cycled ventilators, such as the 'Oxylog' and 'AutoVent 2000', provide variable control of ventilation frequency and minute volume. They are most valuable in confined spaces, especially in rescues involving toxic fumes.

Malleable rubber face masks are most commonly used with resuscitators and there are many varieties of masks available. Regardless of the type of mask in use in your service, the technique of establishing a good seal to the patient's face and the maintenance of the airway are the critical factors. The correct grip will overcome problems of leaks as well as airway control (Fig. 5.13). Frequent practice is an essential element in the maintenance of effectiveness of these vital skills.

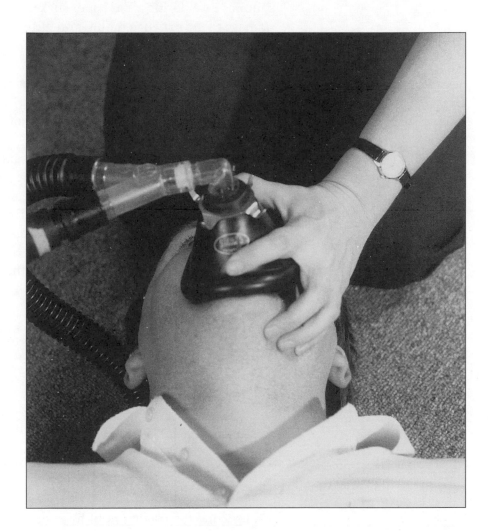

Fig. 5.13 The correct grip for placing a ventilator face mask facilitates gentle pressure and ensures an effective seal.

5

TASKS

1. Assemble a bag-mask ventilator *Use procedure for own equipment*
2. Apply a ventilator mask to a patient's face   260
3. Ventilate a patient using a bag-mask ventilator   261
4. Ventilate a patient using a bag-mask ventilator with oxygen reservoir   261
5. Assemble a demand valve ventilator, or a soft bag rebreathing ventilator   *Use procedure for own equipment*
6. Ventilate a patient using a demand valve ventilator, or a soft bag rebreathing ventilator   262–263

A FEW WORDS ON SUCTION

In Chapter 2 the use of suction in airway management was raised and it was suggested that this technique be limited to removing small volumes of fluids only. Large volumes should be managed by turning the patient allowing gravity to assist.

Suction apparatus varies from manually operated pumps to electrically driven and oxygen-powered devices. The type of equipment available is of less significance than the technique of suctioning an airway. In the ambulance environment, the use of rigid suction tools requires care. Using a Yankauer sucker in a mobile vehicle may cause damage to the patient's mouth and further complicate the airway. Soft suction catheters are safer and equally as effective.

The insertion of any suction tool into a patient's mouth should always be performed under direct vision. Never blindly insert a catheter as you may cause damage. Use a laryngoscope as a lighted spatula to assist in both introducing the sucker and checking the upper airway.

The sucker should be inserted gently and 'swept' across the mouth or throat, withdrawing at the same time. The technique is repeated until the airway has been sufficiently cleared of fluid. Remember that solid debris cannot be suctioned out and requires manual removal. The tip of the sucker should be periodically rinsed with small amounts of water to reduce blockage, but if it becomes obstructed replace it with a new catheter immediately rather than waste time attempting to clear the obstruction.

KNOWLEDGE CHECK

Hypoxia

19. Describe what is meant by the term 'hypoxia'.

20. What are the 2 groups of causes of hypoxia?

21. Describe the 3 clinical features of hypoxia.

22. Describe the treatment of hypoxia.

Respiratory status

23. What are the 3 elements of the respiratory cycle?

24. What is the range of normal respiratory rate?

25. What are the 9 points of the respiratory status assessment?

Oxygen therapy

26. What are the 7 safety precautions for the storage and handling of oxygen?

27. What oxygen flowrate is normally required using a face mask for acutely ill patients?

28. What is the maximum flow rate of oxygen, using a nasal cannula?

Turn to page 300 to check your answers.

THE CLINICAL PROBLEM OF ASTHMA

One of the most common respiratory problems encountered is asthma, a reversible small airway disease, triggered by a wide range of factors, and resulting in bronchial hyper-reactivity. Pathologically, there are three elements:

- Bronchospasm—constriction of the muscular wall of the bronchioles
- Mucousal oedema—swelling of the mucous membrane lining the intima of the bronchioles
- Mucous plugging—thick plugs of sputum obstruct the lumen of the respiratory bronchioles.

In the emergency environment, the only part of this pathology that can be treated pharmacologically is the bronchospasm.

5

TRIGGER FACTORS

Allergy—a frequent cause of episodes of asthma in children and young adults. This may be seasonal, resulting from hypersensitivity to pollens and may be accompanied by hay fever. Close contact with animals usually causes immediate provocation and further reaction several hours later. House dust mite is the most common sensitivity in all age groups. Some people are sensitive to foods such as fish and nuts.

Exercise—transient episodes in children may follow vigorous exercise (e.g., running and jumping) but are less common in adults. Swimming rarely provokes asthma.

Infection—especially upper respiratory tract infection frequently precedes the onset of severe asthma.

Chemicals—colouring agents, such as tartrazine, and flavour enhancing additives to foods, such as MSG, as well as sulphur dioxide used as a food preserver, may provoke attacks. There is also a variety of substances encountered in industry which are recognised as provoking asthma. Recently, atmospheric changes have been linked as a probable trigger factor.

Psychological factors—emotional stress, anxiety and fear may not directly precipitate an episode of asthma, but can exacerbate the effect.

RESPIRATORY CHANGES IN ASTHMA

The construction of the bronchioles, which are muscular tubes, rather than the more rigid, cartilaginous structures of the larger bronchi, enables a variation in their calibre (by dilatation or constriction). The muscular nature means that the calibre will be restricted if the muscle or mucosa is antagonized.

The patient describes a feeling of shortness of breath (dyspnoea) and is usually sitting upright concentrating on breathing. Speech is often difficult as the patient fights to breathe.

Breath sounds in most cases are audible. Expiratory wheeze or cough are normally present, but not all asthmatics wheeze. In mild cases, the main symptom may be cough, with wheeze more evident in intermediate stages. In severe cases, where the patient is unable to generate enough air movement, the wheeze may not be audible. However, all that wheezes is not asthma. Severe allergic reactions and foreign body obstructions in the lower airway may also produce wheeze. Therefore the assessment must be made on other factors, not only breath sounds.

As the small airways become constricted due to bronchospasm, oedema and plugging, the respiratory cycle becomes less rhythmic. Significantly, the respiratory rate increases and a prolonged expiratory phase is evident as the patient attempts to exhale forcefully. Breathing effort changes, with marked chest/abdominal movements and intercostal retractions as the patient uses accessory muscles to improve tidal air movement. In severe respiratory distress, tracheal tugging may be evident.

The changed respiratory cycle and subsequent reduction in tidal movement leads to a mis-match between pulmonary ventilation and diffusion, between alveolar air and pulmonary capillary blood. The result is hypoxia, evidenced by tachycardia, anxiety, pallor and, in severe cases, cyanosis and an altered conscious state.

In severe asthma episodes, the patient is exhausted from the fight to breathe and can appear quite calm. This is often the dangerous stage. Faint breath sounds may indicate complete or nearly complete bronchiole obstruction and inadequate ventilation or both. An altered conscious state and bradycardia may suggest impending respiratory arrest due to inspiratory muscle failure, but is often unpredictable.

Summary of respiratory assessment

	Normal	Asthma
General appearance	Calm, quiet	Distressed, anxious, fighting to breathe, exhausted
Speech	Clear, steady	Difficult, often unable to speak
Breath sounds	Usually quiet	Cough and expiratory wheeze
Respiratory rate	12–16	>20
Respiratory rhythm	Regular, even cycles	Prolonged expiration
Breathing effort	Little, with small chest movement	Marked chest movement, accessory muscles, intercostal retractions, tracheal tugging
Pulse rate	60–80	>100 <60 a late sign in severe cases
Skin	Pink	Pale, sweaty, cyanosed
Conscious state	Alert	Altered

5

MANAGEMENT

In pre-hospital care, as stated earlier, it is possible only to treat the problem of bronchospasm. First order management requires the use of oxygen to deal with the problem of hypoxia and a bronchodilator to ease the effect of the bronchospasm. However, an equally important part of management is calming the patient.

By the time an ambulance responds, the patient has usually spent a considerable amount of time and energy trying to cope with breathing and using prescribed medications. In this exhausted state, the last thing the patient wants to hear is an ambulance officer saying 'Just relax, lean back against the pillow and rest.' This is probably what the patient would like to do most of all, but obviously cannot, so don't speak such pointless words of 'reassurance'.

Asthmatic patients tend to find breathing more easily managed if they can lean forward and rest their arms or elbows on something solid. Don't ask the patient to move, move the patient to minimise further effort. Keep questioning to a minimal level to reduce the need for long verbal responses. Establishing the problem and proceeding with the treatment in a quiet, logical manner is far more reassuring.

Peak expiratory flow (PEF) meters are used by many asthma sufferers to measure and record variations in expiratory efficiency. This record is of value in identifying trends towards episodes of the disease. The use of PEF meters in prehospital care may be suitable for determining critical deficiency, but caution should be taken in making judgements based on one measurement. Many asthmatics record low PEF readings but are not necessarily in danger. The 9-point respiratory status assessment is far more significant in determining the need for respiratory support than a single PEF measurement.

Having completed an assessment of respiratory status and established the need for bronchodilator therapy, firstly administer oxygen via an aerosol mask at 8 litres per minute flow rate. If the patient has any evidence of chronic obstructive airways disease, carefully observe the patient for indications of respiratory depression. However, the acute problem of hypoxia is the primary consideration and the use of high flow oxygen should not be withheld.

The most commonly used bronchodilator in pre-hospital care is salbutamol (see page 204 for pharmacology). The drug is administered via a nebuliser, and given the problem of hypoxia, it is more appropriate to use oxygen at the 8 litre per minute flow rate. High flow rates will also achieve a fine mist. The dosage of salbutamol will vary

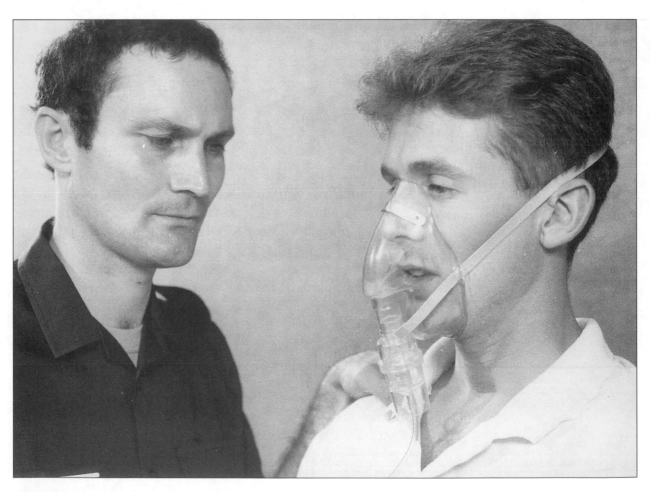

Fig. 5.14 Administering salbutamol using a nebuliser. Make sure that the patient breathes through the mouth.

from service to service, but is usually of the order of 0.2-0.25%. Salbutamol is diluted normally from a stock solution of 0.5% by mixing with normal saline. Pre-mixed nebules of 0.1% and 0.2% are now commonly used.

The most frequently used method of administration is via an aerosol face mask (Fig. 5.14). This mask differs from normal oxygen masks in that the exhaust ports on the sides of the mask are much larger and the adaptor ring at the base is designed to connect a nebuliser. An alternative method of administration, preferred by some patients, is the use of a T-piece tube.

The administration of nebulised salbutamol is best commenced at the scene and continued during transport to the emergency department, rather than waiting for an effect at the scene. The patient will require further management of the oedema and plugging elements of the disease, or often more definitive bronchodilator therapy. Undue delay at the scene is inappropriate and may cause unnecessary distress to the patient or delay urgent intervention of this potentially time critical patient.

Nebulised salbutamol should be used as an in-transit drug.

In the event of the asthmatic patient becoming unconscious or in respiratory arrest, artificial ventilation with oxygen may be life saving. High pressure positive pressure ventilation at a low rate (2-4 litres per minute) and a long expiratory phase is the best pattern. Care should be taken to avoid the possibility of a spontaneous pneumothorax, but it is a rare occurrence.

Status asthmaticus is a prolonged and severe attack, which does not respond to normal treatment. Breath sounds are inaudible because of grossly diminished air movement. The patient is exhausted and relies prominently on the use of accessory muscles in the fight to breathe.

Status asthmaticus is 'time critical' and the management must be directed towards rapid treatment and transport to the emergency department. Medication enroute to hospital is the same as that for acute asthma, but sodium bicarbonate IV may be necessary to correct severe acidosis.

TASKS

CHRONIC OBSTRUCTIVE AIRWAYS DISEASE (COAD)

COAD is a broad term referring to a group of long-standing respiratory disease processes which cause obstruction to the airways and reduced alveolar ventilation. Chronic bronchitis and emphysema are the two most commonly encountered problems in the pre-hospital care environment.

Chronic bronchitis

Chronic bronchitis is an inflammatory disease which causes a narrowing of the bronchial tree. Pathologically, the principal defect is enlargement and over-activity of the mucous secreting glands, resulting in excessive sputum production and a chronic cough. The disease may be due to viral or bacterial infections, air pollution, dust and fumes, and of note, cigarette smoke. Clinically, the patient presents with dyspnoea, a productive cough, wheeze and a prolonged expiratory phase. Cyanosis may be evident in late, severe stages.

Emphysema

Emphysema, commonly accompanied or preceded by chronic bronchitis, is the loss of elastic recoil of lung tissue which results in enlargement of the alveoli. During the expiratory phase, this loss of elasticity causes compression and further collapse of the smaller airways, trapping air in the alveoli. The emphysemic patient must work hard at expiration and this increases the body's energy expenditure rate and breathing effort.

Pursed-lip breathing and the use of accessory muscles is a feature of the breathing effort as the patient attempts to breathe out more forcefully and completely. This breathing pattern and the airway distension eventually causes the chest to become barrel shaped. Cyanosis is a second feature of severe emphysema, due to hypoxia as a result of the mismatch between ventilation and gas exchange in the alveoli.

Alveolar hypoventilation results in carbon dioxide retention in the blood (hypercapnia), which has little effect in mild forms of the disease process, due to the compensatory mechanisms of bicarbonate ion retention and excretory processes of the kidney. However, in severe obstruction in the late stages of the process, severe hypoxia and hypercapnia are present.

Earlier in this chapter, mention was made of the medullary and peripheral chemoreceptors. Their role in the detection of changes in PO_2, PCO_2 and of pH changes in the blood, initiates respiration necessary to maintain homeostasis. The medullary chemoreceptors, which provide the more important stimulus to breathe, are primarily stimulated by an increase in carbon dioxide. The emphysemic patient tends to have permanently elevated levels of carbon dioxide, which causes an acclimatisation of the medullary chemoreceptors.

The peripheral chemoreceptors now provide the main stimulus to breathe and this forms the basis of the concept called the 'hypoxic respiratory drive'. Hypoventilation, and the resultant metabolic acidosis from tissue hypoxia, then produces an exacerbation of the hypercapnic state, which may give rise to a potentially fatal acidosis.

The assessment of the emphysemic patient is made on the nine-point respiratory status assessment criteria, (see page 85 and practical skill guide, page 264) but in order to judge exacerbation, the patient's current respiratory status should be compared with the patient's 'normal' status (long term COAD patients frequently display cyanosis, tachycardia and a degree of dyspnoea as a normal state).

This information then becomes important when considering the use of oxygen therapy. Chronic pulmonary emphysemic patients are often able to tolerate a PO_2 as low as 55 mmHg without showing significant signs of hypoxia, and are therefore compensating and maintaining reasonable homeostasis. However, the patient who presents with severe hypoxia requires oxygen therapy for the rapid reversal of the state.

MANAGEMENT

5

The method of choice for administering oxygen is via a Venturi mask —initially at 28%. However, a nasal cannula, at a flow rate of 2 litres per minute will give an equally effective oxygen flow at 28%. If there is no increase in respiratory rate after 3 minutes, the flow rate should be increased by 1 litre per minute, which will deliver a 32% oxygen concentration. Further 1 litre per minute increments may be continued every 3 minutes, up to a maximum of 6 litres per minute, providing there is no decrease in respiratory rate. If the respiratory rate decreases at any stage with increases of oxygen level, the flow rate should be reduced by 1 litre per minute and maintained at this level until arrival at the emergency department. Respiratory status and heart rate should be monitored every 3 minutes to monitor hypoxic effects and acidotic development.

The aim of pre-hospital management is to control the hypoxia and hence, acidosis, rather than treat the cause of the hypoxia.

THE PROBLEM OF PULMONARY OEDEMA

Pulmonary oedema is commonly associated with left ventricular failure following acute myocardial infarction (AMI) and as such is usually discussed in cardiac related disorders. However, there are other causes of fluid shift into the alveoli which impairs their function. Inhaled irritants and toxic fumes as well as near-drowning and some forms of drug overdose (e.g., heroin) may cause pulmonary oedema.

When the mucous membrane lining the airways is antagonised by irritant substances, the mucous producing glands secrete fluid as a means of 'protection' and removal of the irritant. If the alveolar sacs are antagonised or a foreign substance causes fluid to shift across the diffusion membrane due to an osmotic response (i.e., a fluid shift from a weaker solution to a stronger solution) the fluid will accumulate in the alveoli. This presence of fluid in the alveoli is called pulmonary oedema. In the case of near-drowning, in particular in salt water, blood serum enters the alveoli because of the osmotic effect of the aspirated salt water in the alveoli. However, in the case of toxic fumes, chemical pulmonary oedema is thought to occur through damage to the pulmonary capillary walls, which allows leakage of fluid into the alveoli.

The effect is that of severe restriction of gas exchange across the diffusion membrane, and resultant hypoxaemia. In effect, the patient is drowning in his or her own body fluids. As the fluid volume increases, severe dyspnoea develops and frequently haemoptysis (coughing up frothy, blood-stained sputum). Where pulmonary oedema is due to heart failure following AMI, valvular disease or hypertension, venous congestion in the neck is a significant feature. This is a result of the backlog of blood in the pulmonary network. Further discussion of heart failure can be found in Chapter 6.

MANAGEMENT

Management is aimed at decreasing the patient's oxygen demands and increasing the oxygen level in the alveoli. High flow oxygen and a comfortable sitting posture, along with reassurance and encouragement to slow down respiratory movements is the first order treatment. If the patient presents with wheezy breathing, suggesting some constriction of the respiratory bronchioles, nebulised salbutamol may help improve the air pathway.

KNOWLEDGE CHECK

The problem of asthma

29. Define the term 'asthma'.

30. What are the three elements of the pathology of asthma?

31. Which element of the pathology of asthma can be treated pharmacologically in the pre-hospital care environment?

32. Describe the respiratory changes in asthma.

COAD

33. What is COAD?

34. Describe the pathology of emphysema.

35. List the clinical features of the emphysemic patient.

36. What is the oxygen therapy regime indicated for the management of emphysema?

Pulmonary oedema

37. Describe what is meant by the term 'pulmonary oedema'.

38. Describe the management of pulmonary oedema in pre-hospital care.

Turn to page 301 to check your answers.

5

CASE HISTORY

It is a cold and wet Saturday afternoon, but the shift has been quiet. You and your partner are enjoying the telecast of the football match and a hot cup of coffee, when the despatcher calls:

Respond to 27 Highpoint Drive, Northfield. In a shed at the rear of the premises, a male patient, collapsed, believed as a result of motor exhaust fumes. Emergency response on case number 109 at 1538 hours.

Traffic is light, but heavy rain and slippery road conditions increases your response time to 13 minutes. On arrival, a middle aged man directs you to the patient and explains that he found his 28 year old son in the shed, unconscious on the floor, near the rear of the car. The doors were closed and the car engine was running. He dragged the son to the doorway, placed him on his side and covered him with a tarpaulin to protect him from the rain.

1. **What initial assessment would you make and why?**

2. **What immediate treatment would you commence?**

The father tells you that the patient was still breathing when he was discovered, but it was shallow and there was little chest movement. The vital signs survey reveals:

- *Responding to pain stimulus*
- *Heart rate 116 weak and regular*
- *Respiratory rate 22 prolonged expiratory phase and audible wheeze*
- *Blood pressure 95 systolic*
- *Capillary refill <2 seconds*
- *Skin is cold and clammy. The patient's clothing is wet despite the tarpaulin.*

3. **What judgements do you make from the vital signs?**

4. **Is the patient time critical?**

5. **What further treatment would you consider?**

You continue treatment and load for transport to hospital. In transit, you take the vital signs again, 15 minutes after the initial assessment:

- *Responding to verbal stimulus*
- *Heart rate 100 weak, but improving*
- *Respiratory rate 20 wheeze diminished*
- *Blood pressure 105 systolic*
- *Skin cool to touch and shivering evident.*

6. What is your on-going treatment of the patient during transit to hospital?

7. What information would you provide to the triage nurse on arrival at the emergency department?

Using your patient care record, complete the documentation for the case.

(Answers on page 301)

FURTHER READING

Anon 1989 Respiratory care handbook. Springhouse Corporation, Springhouse

Clark T, Rees J 1985 Practical management of asthma. Methuen, Sydney

McPherson S P 1985 Respiratory therapy equipment. Mosby, St Louis

5

CHAPTER 6
Of perfusion status

The most common problem encountered in pre-hospital care is chest pain of cardiac origin. This chapter centres around cardiovascular disturbances to homeostasis and the management of perfusion disorder. Pain and pain assessment is included as a preliminary to the study and management of cardiac related pain. Likewise haemorrhage and the shock state, along with trauma implications are covered. Basic electrophysiology introduces the essentials of cardiac monitoring and defibrillation as an extension to the first order treatment procedures.

Topics covered

The heart at a glance
The blood vessels
Perfusion status assessment
The problem of pain
The problem of chest pain
Cardiac arrest
The normal ECG
Life threatening dysrhythmia
The shock process
Intravenous therapy (IVT)
The problem of heart failure
A few words on the problem of trauma
Burn injury

6

Aim

To develop an understanding of the cardiovascular system and skills in managing disorders of perfusion status

Learning plan

1. Read each segment of the text information
2. Supplement reading in anatomy and physiology with a more comprehensive text
3. Check your understanding using the knowledge checks
4. Practise the skills using the skills guides as a reference to check your competence

Consider the strenuous muscle activity in running or other forms of hard exercise. When muscles are used for long periods, high levels of nutrients and oxygen are essential. Good perfusion of the muscles requires an efficient pump (the heart) and a transport network (the blood vessels). Likewise, neutralisation and removal of waste materials (via the blood vessels) is essential to ensure continuous muscle function. The heart and blood vessels constantly change body fluids which maintains a fresh state within those fluids.

If the efficiency of the pump is impaired, or failure of the blood vessels to transport nutrients and oxygen adequately to the muscles occurs, homeostasis is compromised and a state of poor or inadequate perfusion exists.

THE HEART AT A GLANCE

The heart's function is to pump blood rich in oxygen and nutrients to all cells of the body and recycle de-oxygenated blood through the lungs for removal of waste gases. This is achieved by two separate cycles of circulation, the heart acting as a double pump.

The size of the heart is roughly about that of the owner's fist; the heart weighs approximately 250 g in an adult (Fig. 6.1). It is located in the mediastinum and is an inverted cone shape with the apex to the left of the midline, resting on the diaphragm, at the level of the 5th intercostal space. The base of the heart is level with the 3rd rib.

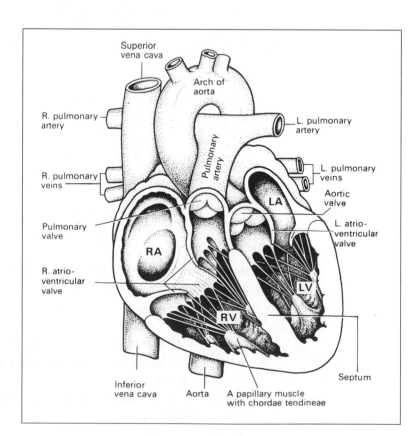

Fig. 6.1 Cross-section showing the interior structures of the heart. (Reproduced with permission from Wilson K J W 1990 Ross & Wilson: Anatomy and physiology in health and illness, 7th edition. Churchill Livingstone, Edinburgh)

The heart wall consists of three layers:

- Endocardium—the smooth innermost layer, folds of which form the heart valves
- Myocardium—the thick muscle layer
- Pericardium—the outermost layer which forms also the pericardial sac enclosing the heart.

The double pump capability is created by the heart being divided into two sides by a thick muscular wall (septum). The left side of the heart provides the pumping force for the systemic (or body) circulation, while the right side maintains the pulmonary circulation. Each side consists of two chambers:

- Atria—collecting chambers for blood returning the lungs (left atrium) and from the body (right atrium)
- Ventricles—pumping chambers to supply bloodflow systemically (left ventricle) and to the lungs (right ventricle).

Non-return valves between the atria and ventricles ensure that the blood flow is in one direction only. Likewise, valves in the *aorta* and *pulmonary artery* prevent blood from returning to the ventricles after ventricular contraction.

CORONARY CIRCULATION

The myocardium needs its own blood vessels to provide oxygen and nutrients and removal of waste materials. The *coronary arteries* (Fig. 6.2 on page 98) are the first branches of the aorta and arise immediately above the aortic valve. After passing through the capillary network in the myocardium, the blood drains into the *cardiac veins* and finally into the coronary venous sinus for return to the right atrium. Because the coronary circulation is constricted during the contraction phase of the cardiac cycle (systole), myocardial blood flow occurs during the resting phase (diastole). Therefore, if the period of diastole is short, blood supply to the heart muscle will be reduced (myocardial ischaemia). Thus, a fast heart rate (tachycardia) will result in reduced pump efficiency and resultant inefficiency in cardiac output.

Another feature of the double pump capability is that both upper chambers (atria) contract in unison and, likewise, the ventricles or lower chambers. The amount of time taken for each contraction and the period of rest is called a cardiac cycle (Fig. 6.3 on page 98). Given an 'average' adult male, with a heart rate of 75 beats per minute, the total time for one beat is 0.8 seconds. That is:

- Atrial systole   =   0.1 seconds
- Ventricular systole =   0.3 seconds
- Cardiac diastole   =   0.4 seconds

The time intervals of both atrial and ventricular systole remain relatively constant. Therefore the variation of rate in heart beat influences the time interval of diastole.

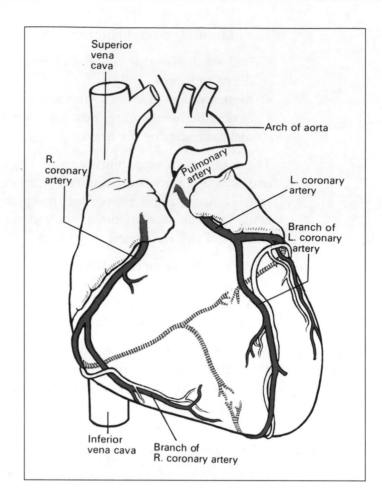

Fig. 6.2 The surface of the heart showing the coronary arteries. (Reproduced with permission from Wilson K J W 1990 Ross & Wilson: Anatomy and physiology in health and illness, 7th edition. Churchill Livingstone, Edinburgh)

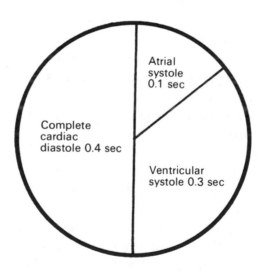

Fig. 6.3 Diagram showing the stages of one cardiac cycle. (Reproduced with permission from Wilson K J W 1990 Ross & Wilson: Anatomy and physiology in health and illness, 7th edition. Churchill Livingstone, Edinburgh)

THE ELECTRICAL CONDUCTION SYSTEM

Unlike other muscle tissue in the body, if the nerves supplying the heart were severed, the heart would continue to beat. While the heart is under the influence of the nervous system, myocardium itself is capable of contracting rhythmically, independent of outside nervous influence. This is due to the electrical conduction system, formed by specialised masses of tissue, having the inherent ability to harness and coordinate the electrical potential generated in the myocardium (Fig. 6.4).

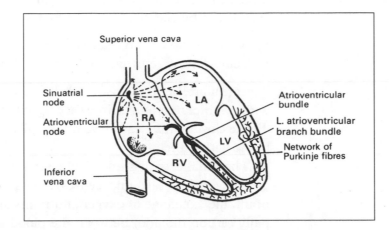

Fig. 6.4 Diagram showing the electrical conduction system of the heart. (Reproduced with permission from Wilson K J W 1990 Ross & Wilson: Anatomy and physiology in health and illness, 7th edition. Churchill Livingstone, Edinburgh)

During the conduction cycle, impulses originating in the 'pacemaker' (sinoatrial node), located in the upper posterior wall of the right atrium, travel throughout the muscle of the atria causing them to contract. At the same time, the impulses stimulate a second node (atrioventricular node), located at the atrioventricular junction of the septum. The relatively slower conduction of the impulses through this node allows time for the ventricles to be filled by the atrial contraction. The wave of excitation travels rapidly through the bundle of His (atrioventricular bundle, located in the septum) and the Purkinje fibres of the ventricular myocardium. This results in the entire musculature of the ventricles contracting in a coordinated manner.

6

KNOWLEDGE CHECK

The heart

1. Describe the location of the heart, using surface anatomy landmarks.

2. What are the three layers of the heart wall?

3. What are the names of the chambers of the heart and what are their functions?

4. Describe the coronary circulation.

5. What are the three elements of the cardiac cycle?

Turn to page 302 to check your answers.

THE BLOOD VESSELS

Before exploring perfusion status and the problems of poor and inadequate perfusion, let's take a quick look at blood vessels. Blood vessels can be classified by their function:

- Arteries—those carrying blood away from the heart
- Veins—those returning blood to the heart.

The great arteries that arise from the heart divide and become smaller, with the thickness and calibre varying with their proximity to the heart. Those close to the heart have thick walls to withstand the pressure of blood within them.

The smallest division of the arteries (arterioles), terminate as *capillaries* which are one cell thickness microscopic tubes. At this point, the exchange of oxygen, nutrients and waste materials (principally carbon dioxide) between the blood and body cells takes place. From the capillaries, blood flows into the smallest veins (venules) and then on into larger veins until returning to the heart via the great veins.

The walls of the arteries consist of 3 coats:

- A smooth inner lining which allows even blood flow—tunica intima
- A bulky layer consisting of elastic connective tissue and smooth (involuntary) muscle which gives the vessel the ability to increase and decrease its diameter (vasodilation and vasoconstriction)— tunica media
- An outer layer consisting of supporting fibrous connective tissue, giving the vessel strength—tunica externa.

The walls of the veins are similar to the arteries, but have a thinner tunica media with less smooth muscle because they carry blood at a low pressure. Veins therefore tend to be less elastic and collapse when they are cut. The veins of the extremities have folds of connective tissue forming valves to prevent backflow and help the blood travel to the heart.

KNOWLEDGE CHECK

The blood vessels

6. **Blood vessels are classified by their function. What are the 2 main types of vessels and their functions?**

7. **What is the name given to the smallest division of the blood vessels?**

8. **What are the names of the 3 layers of the blood vessels?**

9. **Describe the differences between the 2 main types of blood vessels.**

Turn to page 302 to check your answers.

PERFUSION STATUS ASSESSMENT

Perfusion status assessment, in the same manner as the respiratory status assessment, is multifactorial. That is to say that we must gather a wide range of data in order to make an appropriate decision, rather than relying only on one or two observations. While it is obvious that measurements of pulse and blood pressure are good indicators of perfusion, colour, skin temperature and capillary refill provide a more complete clinical picture, together with respiratory evidence and conscious state.

PULSE

As the heart beats, blood is forced into the aorta and pulmonary artery, both of which are already full. Accomodation of this additional volume of blood requires the arteries to expand. The wave of increased pressure travelling along the artery causes alternate expansion and recoil of the vessel, which is described as the pulse. The generation of the pulse wave involves two factors:

- The heart's pumping action. If the blood merely poured out of the heart into the aorta, no pulse would be generated, as the pressure would be constant.
- The elastic property of the artery walls. If vessels were rigid, pressure changes, while still happening, would not generate a palpable pulse. This elasticity ensures a steady and continuous blood flow. Rigidity would result in intermittent rather than continuous flow.

When blood is forced from the heart into the aorta, the first part of this great vessel becomes distended under increasing pressure. It is the only part of the arterial system in which immediate pressure increase occurs. Once sufficient pressure has been reached to overcome the inertia of the blood, the pulse wave is transmitted along the arterial system, growing weaker as it reaches the smaller vessels and finally disappears at the capillary level.

The pulse can be felt at locations where an artery can be held against a bone or firm tissue. The most common sites are:

- The *carotid artery*—at the level of the thyroid cartilage and approximately 4 cm laterally
- The *brachial artery*—located firstly in the medial aspect of the upper arm, in the groove between the biceps muscle and the humerus; and secondly, the medial aspect of the cubital fossa (anterior aspect of the elbow)
- The *radial artery*—in the ventral aspect of the wrist, lateral to the flexor tendon (that is, the thumb side)
- The *femoral artery*—located in the line of the groin at the mid-point between the iliac crest and the symphysis pubis.

6

Palpating the pulse, given that it is produced as a result of each heart beat, can provide information about heart function—that is, its rate, rhythm and strength.

Pulse rates vary with age, exercise, emotion, temperature and disease problems, but commonly accepted ranges per minute are given in the box.

Pulse rates		
• Adult (>12)	=	60—80
• School age child (5 to 12 years)	=	70—120
• Pre-school age child (1 to 5 years)	=	80—130
• Infant (1 to 12 months)	=	100—140

Rates below these ranges (bradycardia) and above (tachycardia) are considered abnormal, but should be considered along with other factors. For example, what of the adult athlete with a resting pulse of 45 per minute?

Rhythm is the regularity of the heart beat. Normal pulse rhythm is regular with evenly spaced beats. Irregular rhythms may be palpated as missed beats, double beats and so on. However, most of the irregularities of the pulse rhythm are innocent, with a few of them being potentially serious. Therefore it is important that the interpretation of the irregularity be made on the patient's total status rather than just the palpation alone.

Strength of the pulse should normally be such that it cannot be too easily obliterated when the pulse site is compressed. Abnormalities of strength include a full, bounding pulse and a weak, thready pulse. While these interpretations are of a subjective nature, we can develop reasonably accurate skill in interpretation if we learn about the strength of a 'normal' pulse.

The final check of the pulse is to 'feel' the artery. A normal artery should feel soft and compliant under your fingers as you palpate the pulse. However, in some circumstances, it may feel hard, wiry, flabby, even tortuous (knotted).

The radial pulse is the most common and convenient site for palpation. In the event of cardiac arrest or if it is difficult or impractical to use the radial site, the carotid pulse is the site of choice. However, in the assessment of the newborn, the brachial pulse is the preferred site because normal sites are often difficult to palpate especially with small musculature in the neck and, in the case of the radial pulse, poorly perfused distal fields.

TASK	Palpate each of the 4 pulse sites (carotid, brachial, radial and femoral) and note the rate, rhythm and strength	267–270

BLOOD PRESSURE

The force exerted by the blood against the walls of the vessels in which it is contained is known as the blood pressure. It is the product of:

- The force of ventricular contraction
- The volume of blood pumped from the heart
- The resistance of the vessels to blood flow.

A liquid will flow only from a region of high pressure to a lower pressure. Therefore, to achieve blood flow, the pressure must be higher in some parts of the circulatory field than in others. The pumping action of the heart creates a pressure gradient between arterial pressure and venous pressure, which is highest in the aorta and at its lowest in the venae cavae.

Blood pressure can be measured against a column of mercury (Hg)—that is to say that the pressure in a blood vessel will exert sufficient force to support a column of mercury to which a scale in millimetres (mm) is applied. For example, if we say that the pressure in the blood vessel is 100 mmHg, this means that the force exerted is sufficient to push a column of mercury up to a level of 100 mm from its base.

During systole, the blood pressure reaches a pressure normally of the order of 120 mmHg and then drops to 80 mmHg during diastole. It is important to remember that although a pulse can be felt only in the arteries, blood pressure exists in all blood vessels. In the venules, the beginning of the venous system, the pressure is about 15 mmHg. This continues to decrease to approximately 5 mmHg at the superior vena cava and is practically 0 mmHg at the right atrium.

Blood pressure is dynamic. That is to say that it changes due to many factors constantly influencing it. Pressure changes will be found from limb to limb and as a result of alteration to posture. Therefore it is important when assessing changes in blood pressure, to ensure that readings are taken on the same limb and in much the same posture.

Other factors affecting blood pressure are similar to those influencing pulse changes:

- Age—blood pressure is lower in children
- Exercise—blood pressure increases in response
- Pain—will usually elevate blood pressure
- Emotion—worry, fear or anxiety will tend to elevate blood pressure
- Bleeding—decrease in blood volume will lead to a decrease in blood pressure
- Drugs and diseases—can either increase or decrease blood pressure.

Commonly accepted systolic ranges are given in the box on page 104.

6

Systolic blood pressure ranges

- Adult (>12)   =   100–160
- School age child (5-12 years)   =   70–90
- Pre-school age child (1-5 years)   =   70–80
- Infants (1-12 months)   =   70

Lower than normal blood pressure is referred to as *hypotension* and higher is *hypertension*. In the emergency environment changes in systolic pressure are more significant than changes in diastolic pressure. For this reason, measuring blood pressure by palpation is the method of choice rather than necessarily auscultating with a stethoscope (Fig. 6.5). Because of the many factors affecting blood pressure, a single isolated reading is usually insignificant. It is also erroneous to rely exclusively on blood pressure, as it is often one of the last observable changes which indicate deterioration in the patient's status. Observation of the other vital signs will show changes often well before blood pressure variations occur.

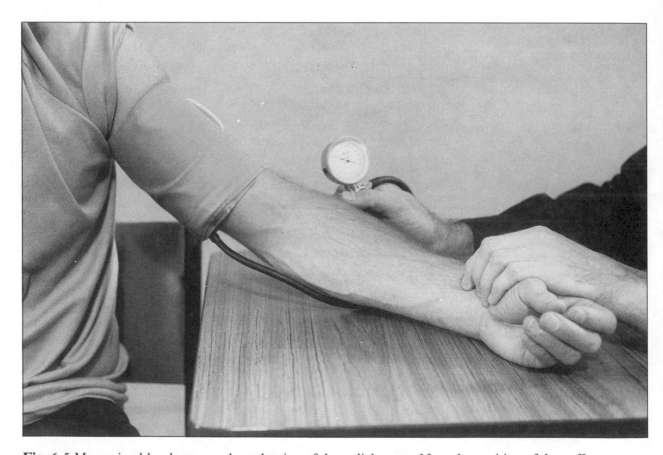

Fig. 6.5 Measuring blood pressure by palpation of the radial artery. Note the position of the cuff.

MEASUREMENT OF BLOOD PRESSURE

Measuring blood pressure needs to be practised frequently to achieve skill in performing the measurement reliably and accurately. Arterial pressure is measured with the aid of a sphygmomanometer which operates by means of either mercury manometer or an aneroid gauge. Aneroid gauges are standardised against a mercury manometer, so that all pressure readings can be expressed in millimetres of mercury.

Accurate recording depends upon several critical details:

- The size of the cuff—too large a cuff will give a falsely low reading and if too small, may give a falsely high reading
- The cuff bladder—should be 20% wider than the diameter of the limb in use
- The cuff must be firmly fitted around a bare limb—too loose a cuff will give a falsely high reading.

TASK   Measure and record a blood pressure by palpation   **271**

SKIN COLOUR AND TEMPERATURE

Usually, when the body is in homeostasis, the periphery (the outer surface) is 'pink' and warm to touch. This is due to adequate perfusion in the peripheral blood vessels (the fine capillaries in the skin) maintaining normal function of the cells.

Look at your own hands as an illustration of normal appearance and the changes when the blood supply is interrupted. To begin with, stretch your arms out in front and check the colour. They should look 'pink' and feel warm. If you have dark skin, check the colour of your nail beds and you should also observe a pink colour. Now raise one arm above your head and hold it there for a minute or so. Bring your arm back to the original position alongside your outstretched arm and compare your hands. The limb (or nailbed) which was elevated appears a pale colour by comparison with the outstretched arm and you may also detect a slight reduction in the temperature of your hand.

Elevating the limb reduces the blood supply to the tissues, draining the blood and therefore 'cooling' the skin. The same result occurs when, following insult to the body, *vasoconstriction* (the shutdown of blood vessels) is brought into action to re-direct available blood volume to vital areas of the body. This is a normal compensatory mechanism of homeostasis, but if sustained, suggests that the body is now struggling to maintain an adequate status. If the deprived tissues do not receive blood and hence oxygen soon, the hypoxic effects will lead to cellular damage. If the degree of hypoxia is severe, cyanosis (a blue colouration in the peripheral areas, commonly the lips, nose, hands and feet) becomes apparent, indicating that urgent treatment with oxygen therapy is required. A pale or cyanotic skin is usually very

6

moist. In patients with dark skin, this colour change may not be easily identified, but if you examine the mucous membranes (inside the mouth or under the eyelids), effective assessment can be made.

Skin *temperature* increases as the blood vessels dilate and decreases as they constrict. The skin is normally warm and slightly moist. The blood vessels dilate in a hot environment or in the case of fever and the skin becomes hot and flushed.

Temperature checking in pre-hospital care does not require the use of a thermometer. While 'feel' is a somewhat subjective assessment, it is quite adequate when used in conjunction with other elements of the check. A simple and useful check with temperature is to compare two different parts of the body—the forehead and tip of the nose, or the illiac crest and big toe. If there is no difference in temperature, then a normal perfusion state exists. A difference in temperature suggests poor peripheral perfusion. This check is performed using the back of the hand, which is more sensitive to temperature variations than the palm—much the same as Mum checking the temperature of baby's bottle.

Observation of skin colour and temperature are then useful indicators of altered perfusion and together with the other elements of the pump and vascular check form an effective evaluation tool.

CAPILLARY REFILL

While we are considering the periphery, an assessment of capillary refill is another element of the perfusion status check. Look at your finger nail beds. They should appear pink. Using the index finger and thumb of one hand, squeeze the nail bed firmly and release it quickly. Watch the colour change and note how long it takes to return to normal.

If adequate perfusion exists, the time taken to return to normal should be less than 2 seconds. Therefore, if the time is more than 2 seconds, it suggests there is a perfusion deficit, giving a further piece of information to use in deciding perfusion status.

OTHER CONSIDERATIONS

Conscious state and breathing, while not essentially part of the direct perfusion picture, are valuable checks. If perfusion is poor, the amount of oxygen available in the body at tissue level is reduced. The outcome is hypoxia, which results in increased respiratory rate and an effort to compensate. If the degree of hypoxia is significant, then the brain may be deprived of oxygen, causing alteration of conscious level.

Combining these elements then provides a broad analysis of perfusion status, upon which judgement may be made about the needs of patient management.

Summary of perfusion status assessment

	Normal	Variations of concern
Pulse	60—80	>100—tachycardia
		<60—bradycardia
Blood pressure	100—160	>160—hypertension
		<100—hypotension
Colour	Pink	Pale, red, cyanosis
Temperature	Warm	Cold and moist/hot and dry

THE PROBLEM OF PAIN

The most common problem encountered in the pre-hospital environment, related to poor or inadequate perfusion, is chest pain of cardiac origin. Before exploring this problem, let's consider the unpleasant sensation called pain.

This abnormal sensation, which may be localised or diffuse, is caused by stimulation of the pain fibres—the specialised peripheral nerve endings—and acts as a physiological protective mechanism. For example, if you touch a hot object, you withdraw your hand rapidly. Apart from causing a few well chosen 'Anglo-saxon' phrases to be uttered, the instant recognition of this unpleasant stimulus and subsequent rapid withdrawal prevents further insult.

However, emotional pain is less tangible and often difficult to manage. Tension, anxiety and fear heighten the response to pain and therefore the approach to management is two-fold. Physical pain is generally easy to combat with the aid of analgesia. A calm, understanding and reassuring approach to the patient will help the emotional factor.

6

PHYSIOLOGY OF PAIN (SIMPLIFIED)

1. The sensory nerves respond to an external stimulus. This might be quite routine in the case of body position or pressure. On the other hand the stimulus may be noxious, such as heat or cold, sharp or blunt.
2. The brain (or spinal cord, in the case of reflex arc function) receives information from the sensory nerves and interprets the stimulus, deciding whether action should be taken.

3. An appropriate reaction normally occurs to relieve the pain—for example:

- A flight response—a tendency to move away from the stimulus
- An immobilisation response—keeping the stimulated area motionless (as seen in rib fracture where the patient tends to guard chest movement to ease the pain).

If the stimulus is overwhelming, collapse may result.

The symptom of pain is an important tool in identifying problem areas and therefore is of great benefit to the medical officer in establishing a diagnosis. In pre-hospital care, the emphasis is on problem identification and management, not diagnosis. However, a thorough pain assessment will help to direct the most appropriate form of treatment.

PAIN ASSESSMENT

When collecting the data for pain assessment, it is important not to overlook relevant information. The mnemonic 'DOLOR' (Latin for pain) is a helpful guide.

Description. It is advisable *not* to ask 'Have you any pain?' or 'Where does it hurt?'- as such approaches may lead to implanting symptoms in the patient's mind. A suitable approach is to ask 'Can you describe your discomfort'. The patient may then respond with 'pressure' or 'tightness', rather than associate these symptoms with pain. You should also ask whether the patient has had this before and whether it is the same, worse or better.

Onset and duration. 'When did it begin? What made it start? Did it start suddenly or come on gradually? What were you doing when it started? Has it been the same since it started or has it changed? How has it changed?'

Location. 'Point with one finger to where you feel the discomfort. Do you feel it elsewhere? Has the feeling stayed in one place or has it moved? Where to?'

Other signs/symptoms. 'Indigestion', nausea, vomiting, sweating, dyspnoea, bleeding, coughing.

Relief. 'Have you taken anything to relieve the feeling?' (food, medicine, drink etc.) Did you do anything to try to relieve it?' (sit up, walk, curl up, lie down etc.) 'Did anything help? Did the feeling return? Was it the same or different?'

It may better serve the patient's interests if the assessment is as brief as possible. Long questioning must not compromise patient care, nor heighten anxiety.

ANALGESIA

The effective relief of pain depends on the two-fold approach mentioned earlier (physical and emotional support). Inhalational analgesics act rapidly and are most suited to the pre-hospital care setting. Constant monitoring of the patient is essential during administration as most analgesics will cause depression of body functions, especially respiratory and conscious status.

Patients suffering from trauma, chest pain or obstetric problems are most likely to need analgesia. Remember that there is no need to give pain relief to patients who, regardless of injury, do not display signs of distress or do not complain of pain. It is also important to remember that pain associated with trauma is relieved by the effective treatment of the injuries. Immobilising fractures, supporting injured regions and posture all assist in the management of pain.

Entonox

A satisfactory and safe inhalational analgesic, Entonox has been used for many years. Stored as a compressed gas in a standard cylinder (colour coded blue, with white shoulders), Entonox is a 50/50 mixture of nitrous oxide and oxygen. Therefore it provides a relatively high concentration of oxygen and because it is relatively odourless, is tolerated by most patients.

The gas is flammable and should be used carefully in rescue incidents where sparks and flames may exist. When exposed to freezing or temperatures below 5°C, the 50/50 proportion is lost, but can be overcome by shaking the cylinder before use.

Entonox acts quickly and does not produce side effects. However, some patients may become drowsy, but return to an alert state once administration is stopped. No masking of physical signs is produced on ceasing administration and it does not cause problems with any subsequent anaesthesia requirements on arrival at the emergency department. It may be given following narcotic analgesia, in which case, the analgesic effect is increased.

Entonox is normally self-administered via a demand valve and mask (Fig. 6.6 on page 110). However, there are some circumstances where the ambulance officer may administer the gas (if the patient has fractures to the upper limbs or if the limbs are trapped). If this is the case, then monitoring conscious status is vital, removing the mask if there is any depression.

Regardless of circumstances, at no time should the valve mechanism be activated by the ambulance officer.

6

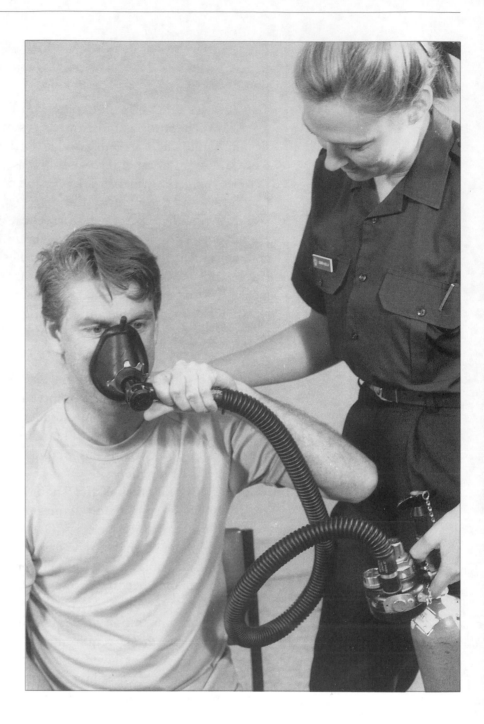

Fig. 6.6 Self-administering Entonox. Make sure the patient does not block the exhaust valve.

Methoxyflurane

Another commonly used inhalational analgesic in pre-hospital care is methoxyflurane (Penthrane). A potent anaesthetic agent, methoxyflurane, when used in conjunction with oxygen, provides rapid pain relief (within 3-5 minutes).

Methoxyflurane can be administered to most patients safely, with the exception of those with severe renal disease or eclampsia. The normal dose is 3ml to a maximum of 6 ml.

Methoxyflurane may produce side effects with overdose (varying degrees of renal disease, which is usually reversible, except in extreme cases). The odour is sweet and strong but tolerated by most patients.

It is often described as similar to 'juicy fruit' chewing gum.

Administration of methoxyflurane is by one of two methods in pre-hospital care.

- Analgiser inhaler—a hand held unit for self administration (oxygen supplementation is required via a nasal cannula)
- In-circuit vaporiser attached to the Oxy-Resuscitator (used extensively in some services).

The use of pharmacological agents in pre-hospital emergency care, not only analgesics but all drugs, requires the consent of the patient and evidence of use must be recorded.

> **ALWAYS REMEMBER YOU OPERATE UNDER THE AUTHORITY OF YOUR SERVICE MEDICAL OFFICER AND USE OF THESE DRUGS OUTSIDE AUTHORISED DUTY IS ILLEGAL**

TASKS

THE PROBLEM OF CHEST PAIN

6

Chest pain is the common mode of presentation of acute myocardial infarction (AMI). (Myocardial refers to heart muscle, and infarction to death.) However, it is important to realise that there are many other causes of chest pain, some of which are not life threatening. Further, the nature of chest pain, especially of non-traumatic origin, is a referred pain—that is to say that where it is felt is not the site of the problem. The answer to this riddle lies in the structure of the nervous system.

Sensory pathways from the organs of the thorax and abdomen join the spinal cord from the region of the first thoracic vertebra (T1) to the second lumbar vertebra (L2). Concentrating on the thoracic pathways, we note that they run from the various organs and structures through a mass called the lateral chain of ganglia. From there, they join the spinal cord via pathways connected to segments from T1 to T5, not necessarily passing directly across the lateral chain of ganglia (see Fig. 6.7 on page 112). The brain, on receiving this sensory stimulus cannot discriminate the precise point of origin. Complicating the interpretation also is the fact that the sensory innervation from the skin of the thorax and upper limbs enters the spinal cord through the same segments. Hence, the pain is usually poorly localised, often diffuse, vague and referred to the skin (see Fig. 6.8 on page 112).

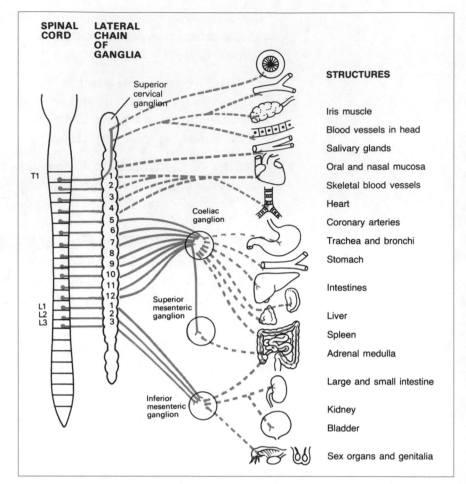

Fig. 6.7 Sensory pathways, including those from the organs of the thorax and abdomen showing common linkages to the spinal cord. (Reproduced with permission from Wilson K J W 1990 Ross & Wilson: Anatomy and physiology in health and illness, 7th edition. Churchill Livingstone, Edinburgh)

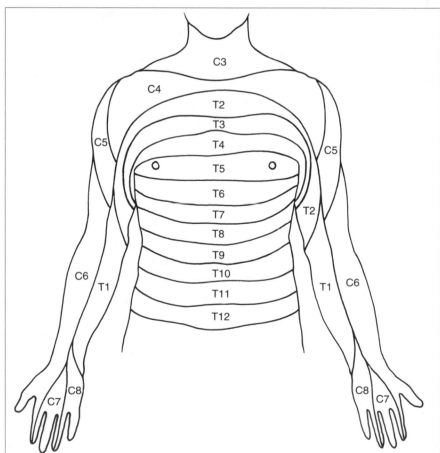

Fig. 6.8 Referred pain is a result of the relationship between the skin and the spinal nerves. The sensory innervation of specific areas of the skin of the thorax and upper limbs is linked to particular segments of the spinal cord.

The approach to all chest pain or discomfort, is to assume AMI until proven otherwise.

The reason is that AMI is the most severe cause of such pain, and the approach applies especially where there is apprehension or general symptoms of a non traumatic and non pleuritic nature.

CORONARY ARTERY DISEASE

Earlier in this chapter, we explored briefly the structure of the heart and in particular, its blood supply—the coronary circulation. We noted that the supply of blood was viable only during the rest phase of the cardiac cycle (diastole) and that if the heart rate increases, the period of rest is reduced, thus limiting the supply of blood to the myocardium. This effect we might refer to as 'natural ischaemia'. But what if it occurs because of unnatural events? Deposits of material may form on the walls of the vessels thus reducing their lumen; 'hardening' of the muscular layer of the vessels may occur, reducing their ability to dilate. These processes form a 'family' of diseases known as *arteriosclerosis*. Atherosclerosis, a common member of this family, is characterised by changes in the intima of arteries, notably the aorta, coronary and cerebral arteries. Accumulation of fatty products, carbohydrates and blood products on the artery walls narrows the vessels reducing blood flow.

Any event that reduces the blood supply to the myocardium (myocardial ischaemia) results in a reduced efficiency of the pump. The effect is, therefore, a reduction in blood supply to the tissues of the body. The brain, monitoring homeostatic balance throughout the body, influences the heart to increase its rate to compensate for the reduction. But, with a reduced blood supply itself, the heart is distressed, which is signalled by the onset of the 'referred' chest pain.

Before we look at the classic pictures of this chest pain, let's consider the risk factors associated with coronary artery disease:

* Age and sex
* Diet and high serum cholesterol
* Hypertension
* Sedentary life-style
* Cigarette smoking
* Family history of heart disease
* Obesity
* Diabetes
* Emotional stress

There is no proof that these and other factors are in themselves the direct cause of arterial disease. However, these factors may contribute to the formation of atheroma and the progression of the disease process.

6

ANGINA

Angina (or more correctly, angina pectoris) is the name given to the distinctive type of chest pain associated with myocardial ischaemia. The onset of the pain is usually precipitated by physical effort or emotional stress and relieved by rest or medication. Duration is characteristically short, but may persist for longer periods, especially if the stimulus for the episode is intensive.

Anginal pain is often described as like a tight belt around the lower chest and may radiate to the neck and jaw, shoulders and arms. Dyspnoea and apprehension are symptoms and the effects of hypoxia and peripheral shutdown completes the general clinical picture.

Patient management involves rest, oxygen therapy and glyceral trinitrate (GTN). GTN is a vasodilator drug, commonly prescribed as a sublingual tablet. Should the pain pattern worsen or fail to be consistently controlled by rest and GTN, then a deterioration of the patient's coronary artery disease is presumed.

ACUTE MYOCARDIAL INFARCTION (AMI)

Severe and prolonged myocardial ischaemia will cause localised death of myocardial tissue. This process is termed acute myocardial infarction.

The majority of AMI are as a result of coronary artery atherosclerosis. The site of tissue death depends on which artery is blocked. The extent of the infarct is determined by the size of the artery obstructed and the capacity of the collateral circulation (secondary vessels) to supply blood to the oxygen deprived area. Pathologically, during the early stages of AMI, there are three zones of tissue damage identified:

- The inner zone consists of an area of irreversible necrosis (destroyed tissue)
- The middle zone where the tissue is injured, but may survive if an adequate circulation can be restored
- The outer zone consists of ischaemic tissue, but will recover unless the ischaemia worsens.

The ultimate size of the infarct depends on the rapidity of onset, the effectiveness of the collateral circulation and the efficiency of early treatment.

The clinical presentation of AMI is similar to that of angina, although the onset of pain tends to be sudden, often during rest. However, this differentiation may not necessarily be accurate, because patients with 'unstable angina' may also experience rapid onset of chest pain with diminishing effort as the disease progresses.

Summary of clinical presentation of chest pain	
Appearance	Pale, cold and sweaty; anxious; apprehensive; dyspnoeic
Pain	Referred across chest wall; may radiate to neck, jaw and arms; nature—a tight belt, vice-like, crushing discomfort
Pulse	Frequently weak and rapid; often irregular
Other	Nausea, sometimes vomiting

MANAGEMENT

Management of the patient with acute chest pain is aimed at reducing the workload on the heart and increasing the oxygen supply to the tissues. Rest the patient in the most comfortable posture and do not move the patient more than is absolutely necessary. Under no circumstances should the patient be walked as this will greatly increase cardiac workload. A calm, reassuring manner is essential to help relieve anxiety and apprehension. Analgesia with high flow oxygen supplement is vital to reduce both the physical and emotional impact of the incident. Transport to the emergency department without delay is required as this problem is potentially time critical. Maintain regular assessments of physiological status (respiratory, perfusion and conscious status), be alert to the possible complications following AMI, and take the appropriate action (Fig. 6.9).

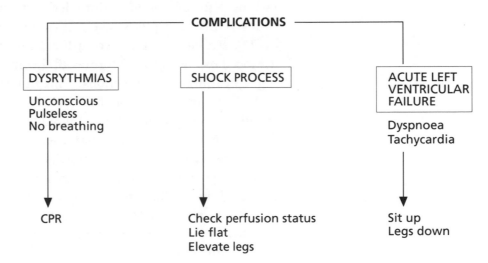

Fig. 6.9 Post AMI complications.

In recent times, new drugs have been developed to reduce the onset of AMI in patients presenting with chest pain of cardiac origin. Antithrombolytic therapy minimises clot formation, thus reducing the incidence of coronary artery obstruction. These drugs are most effective during the first hour of onset of chest pain. However, they are not widely used in the pre-hospital care environment at present, due to cost and the need for careful administration.

CARDIAC ARREST

Cardiac arrest is a common sequel to AMI and is often heralded by a very irregular pulse. Peri-arrest seizure, caused by hypoxia is often seen. The first order management is CPR. Frequently, the underlying cause of arrest is a dysrythmia (changed electrical impulse occurring outside the control of the heart's conduction system). Most commonly the dysrythmia is *ventricular fibrillation* (VF). CPR, while maintaining a forward movement of blood, will have no effect on this dysrythmia. Electrical *defibrillation* is required rapidly because the longer the patient is in VF, the less chance there is of successful reversion to a life sustaining rhythm.

Before considering the management of dysrythmias and in particular, the defibrillation procedure, let's return to the electrical conduction system and explore the electrical picture.

The structure of the myocardium is a specialised form of muscle arranged in a lattice work form with the fibres dividing and recombining, spreading in all directions. This multinucleate mass of merging cells (syncytium) is so tightly bound together that if an impulse stimulates one cell, it will travel rapidly through all the cells. This 'all or nothing' principle means that when the myocardium is stimulated, the whole syncytium contracts. Because the heart consists of two separate syncytiums (atrial and ventricle syncytiums), the contraction phases of the cardiac cycle occur separately. If the impulses stimulating electrical action in the syncytiums are coordinated, then an effective cycle is produced, and at a rate which maintains a constant forward movement of blood to the body tissues.

Consider the effect of an impulse leaving the pacemaker (sinoatrial node (SA node)) and stimulating a complete electrical response across the heart. The impulse spreads in all directions across the atrial myocardium because of its syncytial nature.

As the impulse reaches each cell, an electrical discharge is caused by a change in the polarity of the cell. That is to say that the cell's charge changes from positive to negative through the interaction of sodium ions (negative) and potassium ions (positive). This change is called *depolarisation*. The resultant effect is atrial syncytium contraction.

At the same time, the impulse is conducted to the atrioventricular node (AV node). Because of the dense fibrous nature of the nodal tissue and the AV bundle, the impulse slows, picking up speed again as it passes along the left and right bundle branches. When the impulse reaches the end of the fine Purkinje network, the ventricular syncytium is depolarised, resulting in ventricular contraction.

Following depolarisation, the myocardial cells reform the positive charge, ready for the next cycle of contraction. This reformation of electrical energy is called *repolarisation*.

The frequency of impulses stimulating depolarisation depends on the emissions from the SA node. It has an inherent rate of 60-80 per minute and is the fastest and therefore the dominant pacemaker. Information from the brain, concerning the body's demands for circulatory supply, influence the rate of impulse emission from the SA node.

The AV node will discharge impulses at a rate of 40-60 per minute, and the slowest pacing point of the circuit is the Purkinje fibres, with an inherent rate of 15-40 per minute.

The electrical activity of the heart can be observed by means of an oscilloscope, which will display the different parts of the electrical phase in a regular, repeating pattern. This pattern is called an *electrocardiograph* (ECG).

KNOWLEDGE CHECK

6

Electrical conduction

10. Draw a diagram of the heart and insert the 5 main elements of the conduction path.

11. What is meant by the term depolarisation?

12 What is meant by the term repolarisation?

13. What is the inherent rate of the SA node, AV node and Purkinje fibres?

Turn to page 302 to check your answers.

THE NORMAL ECG

Figure 6.10 shows the normal ECG pattern. Atrial depolarisation is represented by the P wave and is produced by the impulses spreading across the atria. The PR interval represents the time the impulse takes to spread through the AV node and junctional tissue.

Ventricular depolarisation is represented by the QRS complex and is produced by impulses passing through the bundle branches to the Purkinje fibres.

Ventricular repolarisation is represented by the T wave and is the reformation of the electrical charge in the ventricular syncytium during relaxation (or diastole).

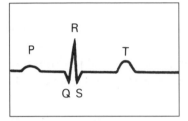

Fig. 6.10 An electrocardiogram of one cardiac cycle. (Reproduced with permission from Wilson K J W 1990 Ross & Wilson: Anatomy and physiology in health and illness, 7th edition. Churchill Livingstone, Edinburgh)

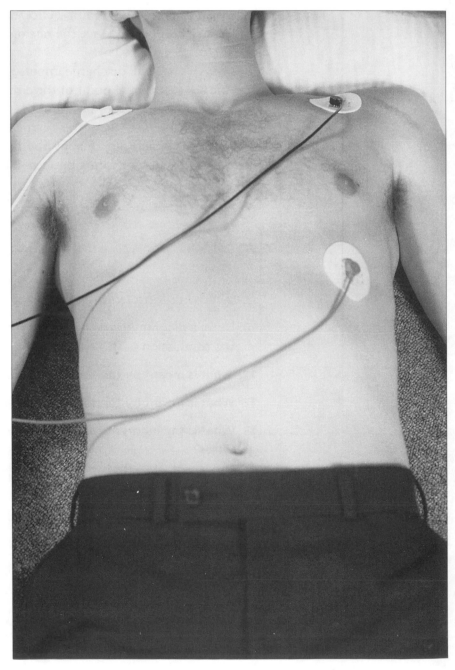

Fig. 6.11 Avoid body hair and bulky muscle when placing electrodes for an ECG.

The normal ECG, consisting of repeating and normal deflections at a constant rate, is called *normal sinus rhythm*. That is, the rhythm created is under the control of the sinoatrial node and is the rhythm expected with normal cardiac function.

An ECG is produced by attaching electrodes to a patient's arms and legs over bony prominences. In the emergency setting, however, the method of choice for monitoring is by placing the electrodes on the patient's chest (Fig. 6.11). A 3-lead attachment is used and the electrodes, which are both colour coded and marked with limb references, are placed on the chest.

Placement of electrodes for ECG

- White (RA (right arm)). Attached to right chest, beneath lateral third of the clavicle
- Black or green (LA (left arm)). Attached to left chest, beneath lateral third of clavicle
- Red (LL (left leg)). Attached to left costal margin, mid-clavicular line.

The correct placement of the electrodes is vital to ensure a clear recording for interpretation. This placement will also become important when we introduce the defibrillation paddles. Avoid areas of excessive hair, because the electrodes will not adhere to the skin correctly, causing a poor signal, which might lead to the rhythm being misinterpreted. Likewise, avoid areas of large muscle mass, as other muscle activity will be amplified and distort the cardiac picture.

6

THE ECG MONITOR/DEFIBRILLATOR

There is a wide variety of ECG monitors and defibrillators in use in pre-hospital care. Nevertheless, they are all similar in function, with the capacity to both monitor cardiac rhythm and provide the means for defibrillation. Arguably the most commonly used unit is the 'Lifepak-5', so let's use that as our example (Fig. 6.12 on page 120). The unit consists of two components:

- The monitor, which provides a visual display and a recording strip
- The defibrillator, which is capable of delivering an output of up to 360 joules.

Accessories are contained within a pouch attached to the unit. These items include:

- A patient cable (3-lead)
- ECG electrodes
- Recording paper
- Gel pads for defibrillating.

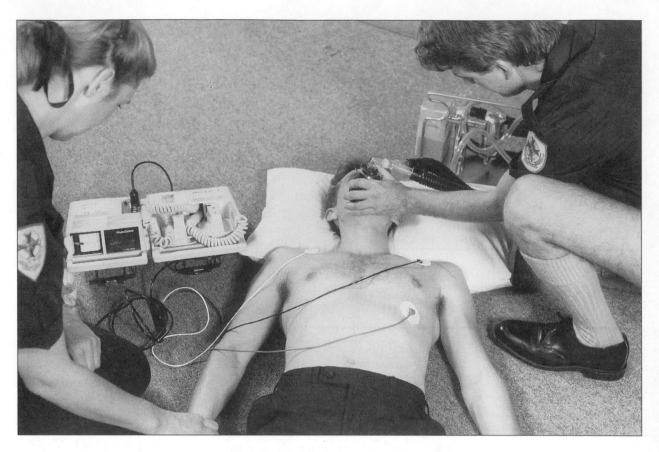

Fig. 6.12 Monitoring an ECG using the Lifepak-5 unit. As part of the management of the chest-pain patient, the monitor should be positioned near enough for ease of viewing and defibrillation.

On the control plate is a lead selector switch, which enables monitoring of the three leads. However, in the emergency setting, lead II is the most relevant, providing all that we need to view.

The ECG paper is marked with a graph grid in millimetres, enabling measurement in amplitude as well as longitude (Fig. 6.13). Longitudinal measurement is of more significance to us, so let's concentrate on that. Given that the speed of the recording is controlled at a normal rate of 25mm per second, the segments of the normal ECG can be timed. Each small square (1mm^2) is equal to 0.04 seconds. The grid is marked with a darker line every 5mm, which therefore represents 0.2 seconds.

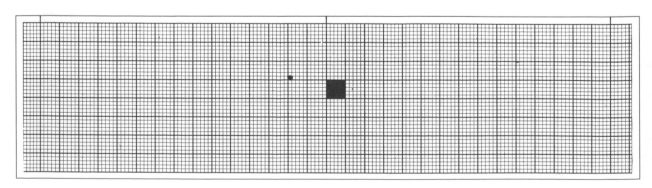

Fig. 6.13 ECG paper showing the grid markings.

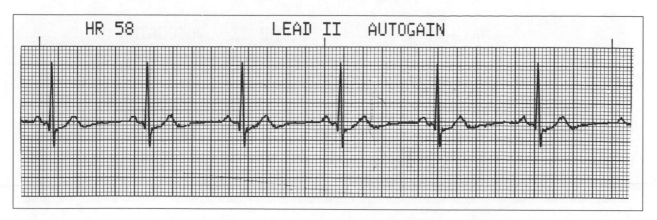

Fig. 6.14 ECG—normal sinus rhythm.

If we now look at the normal ECG in Figure 6.14 we can see that the 'P' wave is of about 2 mm duration, which is 0.08 seconds and the QRS complex about 3 mm, which is 0.12 seconds. We can also see the time delay between the beginning of atrial depolarisation and the beginning of ventricular depolarisation. This is the PR interval and is about 5 mm, or 0.2 seconds. Using these as standard measures of the normal sinus rhythm, abnormal presentations can be interpreted against this information.

Consider the ECG in Figure 6.14. It shows a normal sinus rhythm, with a rate of about 60 per minute. This is arrived at by counting the number of QRS complexes over a 6 second period and multiplying that number by 10, giving the rate per minute.

6

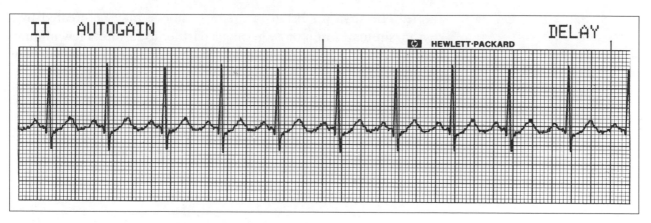

Fig. 6.15 ECG—sinus tachycardia.

Now consider Figure 6.15. It shows a rate of 100 per minute. However, the rhythm is still the same sinus rhythm as we saw before, but the interval between the T wave and the next P wave is decreased. This is a normal variation of sinus rhythm when the heart is required to increase its rate. The ECG shows *sinus tachycardia*—a fast sinus rhythm.

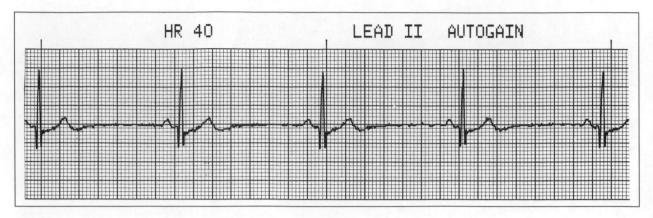

Fig. 6.16 ECG—sinus bradycardia.

If the rate is slowed down (Fig. 6.16), the interval between the T wave and the next P wave is increased. The ECG is otherwise quite normal and shows *sinus bradycardia*—a slow sinus rhythm.

Remember the ECG displays electrical information only. Physical function requires pulse measurement.

TASK

1. Set up an ECG monitor for a lead II recording   277
   Discuss recordings of:
   - Normal sinus rhythm
   - Sinus tachycardia
   - Sinus bradycardia

(Note: The rhythms listed in the tasks above may be created by a rhythm simulator unit or by getting a partner to rest for a few minutes before recording in the case of sinus bradycardia, or exercise for a few minutes before recording in the case of sinus tachycardia.)

LIFE THREATENING DYSRHYTHM

VENTRICULAR FIBRILLATION

As mentioned earlier, the most common lethal dysrythmia following AMI is ventricular fibrillation. This occurs as a result of the injured zone of myocardium becoming an irritable focus, which triggers intermittent and uncontrolled depolarisation of groups of myocardial cells. Because the impulses are rapid, this focus becomes the dominant pacing site, but due to no coordination of the depolarising action, causes the ventricular syncytium to quiver in useless contractions.

The ECG (Fig. 6.17) shows a bizarre, irregular saw tooth pattern, which can only be reversed to a functional rhythm by a counter-shock. This, then, is the purpose of defibrillation or direct current counter-shock (DCCS).

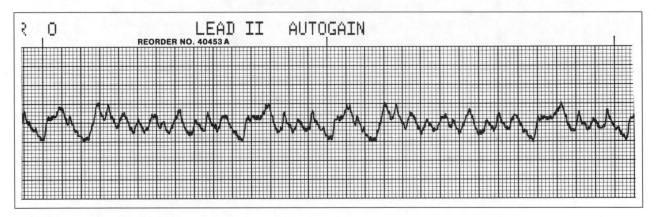

Fig. 6.17 ECG—ventricular fibrillation.

DEFIBRILLATION

The defibrillator is activated by selecting 'paddles' by a switch on the Lifepak-5, or in the case of other units, 'arming' the defibrillator. Gel pads should be placed on the chest sites to aid conduction of the energy and reduce the tendency of burning the skin. The gel pads are placed (Fig. 6.18 on page 124):

- just right of the sternum beneath the clavicle
- below the line of the left nipple, on the mid axillary line.

Place the paddle electrodes on the gel pads, keeping them firm and steady. Charge the defibrillator to the required power setting (normally 200 joules at first). This is done by either dialling the required setting on the paddle control or on the face plate of the monitor.

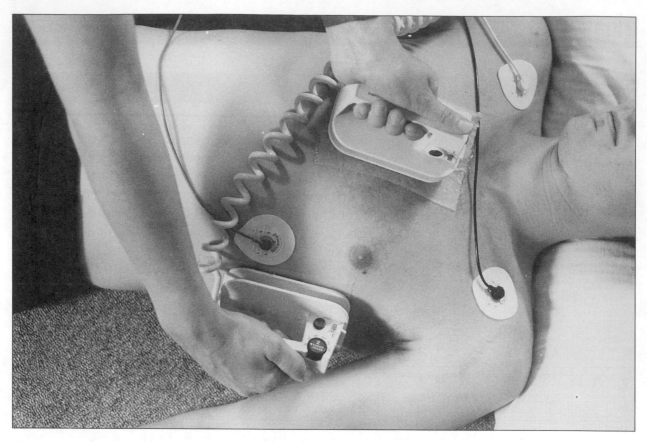

Fig. 6.18 Placement of gel pads and paddles for defibrillation. Make certain that pads and paddles are clear of electrodes and cables.

You must confirm that the rhythm shown on the monitor is VF before defibrillating.

If the patient is in contact with a metal surface, or in water, the energy will be conducted to other objects or persons in contact, or yourself. Physically check the surroundings and it also pays to call 'all clear.'

> **YOU MUST MAKE SURE THAT IT IS SAFE TO DEFIBRILLATE**

The defibrillator is discharged by depressing both paddle switches simultaneously. Re-check the monitor for rhythm change and assess the carotid pulse for cardiac output. Remember that the ECG shows only the electrical picture. The mechanical function of cardiac output may not necessarily be associated with the electrical image. This phenomenon is most commonly caused by 'electromechanical dissociation' or EMD, in which electrical activity is occurring, but physical contraction does not follow.

VENTRICULAR TACHYCARDIA

In Figure 6.19, we observe wide and frequent QRS complexes. This is a fast ventricular rate, but unlike VF, is a coordinated depolarisation within the ventricular syncytium. If this ventricular tachycardia is seen and there is no evidence of output by palpation of the carotid pulse, defibrillation is indicated. However, if the pulse is present, the heart is functioning—albeit with grossly reduced efficiency—and defibrillation must not be attempted.

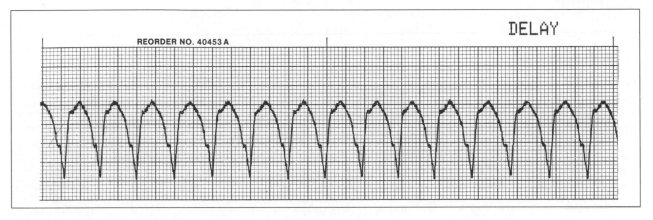

Fig. 6.19 ECG—ventricular tachycardia.

ASYSTOLE

The third lethal arrythmia is asystole, or cardiac standstill. The ECG (Fig. 6.20) shows absence of any discernible complexes and the trace is almost a straight line. Defibrillation in this case may have little effect as an iso-electric presentation (a straight line) suggests that there is little repolarisation in the myocardial cells to sustain a rhythm. However, in some protocols, asystole is defibrillated, but usually following drug therapy to stimulate the myocardium (e.g., adrenaline and isoprenaline).

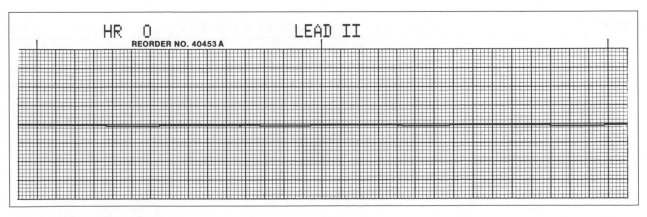

Fig. 6.20 ECG—asystole.

Putting all of this together with the basic life support approach described in Chapter 2, the immediate life support process is complete (see Fig. 6.21).

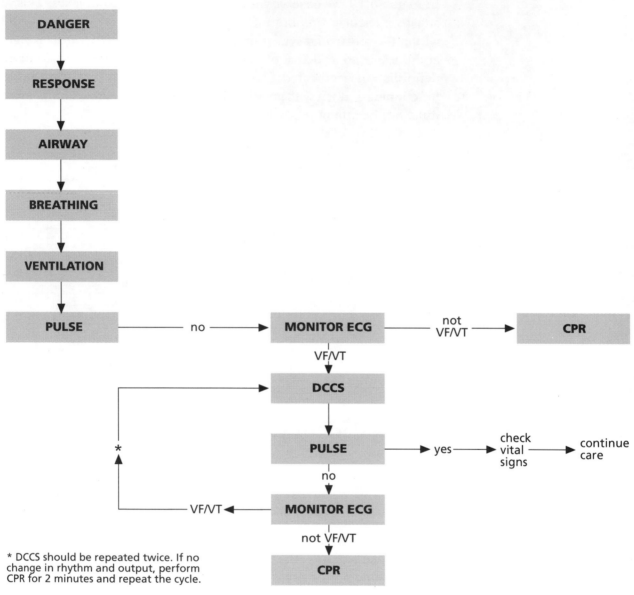

* DCCS should be repeated twice. If no change in rhythm and output, perform CPR for 2 minutes and repeat the cycle.

Fig. 6.21 Defibrillation flowchart.

TASK   Defibrillate a patient presenting with VF/VT   278

It is most important to remember that during the setting up of the monitor/defibrillator, basic life support measures and CPR must be continued. This technology does not stand alone. Basic 'hands-on' skills are the essential cornerstones of this procedure, without which the technology is almost useless.

THE SHOCK PROCESS

The second complication associated with chest pain, and indeed almost every insult to the body, is the shock process. The word 'shock' is imprecise and a simple definition is not readily achieved, because it is not a single entity with a specific cause or treatment. The term 'shock process' is an attempt to understand the body's struggle for survival in adverse situations and the preservation of its most vital functions.

The overall body response to insult is a complex series of reactions to restore and maintain adequate tissue perfusion and circulating blood volume. Causes can be broadly categorised as fluid loss (absolute or relative) or of cardiac origin (cardiogenic).

Absolute fluid loss. This involves loss of fluids (blood, plasma, water and minerals) from the vascular and/or cellular environment, for example, blood loss, due to external bleeding or internal bleeding (both revealed and concealed) or plasma, water and mineral loss, due to burn injury or dehydration.

Relative fluid loss. There is no physical loss from the body, but a shift of fluid from the vascular bed. Examples are 'fainting' (syncope) or a vasovagal response, causing 'pooling' of blood in an area of the vascular system; anaphylaxis (an 'explosive' response to foreign proteins); overwhelming infections, causing fluid shift into tissues. Absolute and relative fluid loss categories might also be described as 'hypovolaemic shock'.

Cardiogenic. This involves failure of adequate perfusion of fluids, due to the inadequacy of the heart as a pump. For example, following AMI, the damaged myocardium can no longer effectively keep pace with the body's demands for circulatory supply. Pain and emotional influences of AMI also impact on pumping efficiency following AMI.

There is also a *multifactorial category* to consider when discussing shock. A fracture of a long bone, e.g., the femur, results in absolute fluid loss (bleeding into tissues) and the effects of pain and emotion impinge on pump function and fluid shift in the vascular bed.

6

STEPS IN THE PROCESS

Using the example of a slow continuing bleeding event, let's analyse each of the steps in the process.

1. Event—slow continuing haemorrhage

The rate of blood loss is not rapid. The blood loss cannot be controlled by simple means. The escape of blood from the blood vessels is either external or internal.

There are many causes of this slow continuing haemorrhage. For example, a small tear in the aorta, spleen or liver; a bleeding gastric ulcer; a simple fracture of a long bone (femoral shaft). Therefore an adequate *history* of the event is essential in determining the cause of the bleeding.

2. Blood loss—decreased venous return, decreased cardiac output

Body circulation is a 'closed system'. The same volume returns to the heart (venous return (VR)) which is pumped out of the heart (cardiac output (CO)).

If blood is lost from the vessels, venous return decreases. If venous return decreases, then it is also true that cardiac output decreases.

3. Decrease detected by receptors—action initiates compensation

In the walls of the great arteries (aorta and arteries) there are pressure receptor cells. These receptors monitor the blood pressure and provide the brain, via sensory nerve pathways, with information about changes in blood pressure. As blood loss occurs and cardiac output (and venous return) decreases, the blood pressure falls. The brain initiates a compensatory action to return cardiac output to normal. This is done by increasing both the heart rate and the stroke volume (the volume pumped from the ventricles with each ventricular contraction). Vasoconstriction enables the stroke volume to be increased. An increased heart rate is tachycardia.

4. Tachycardia

As the blood loss continues, the heart rate rises to maintain cardiac output. However, the effectiveness of the pump decreases once the rate exceeds about 140-180 beats per minute. Any heart rate greater than 120 per minute is considered to be a serious, if not critical, sign. Let's assume that the normal heart rate (HR) is the middle of the range (60-80). The stroke volume (SV) is also middle of the range (70-90 ml). The cardiac output (CO) is the product of heart rate and stroke volume:

HR x SV = CO
i.e., 70 x 80 = 5600 ml/min.

As blood loss occurs, the volume of blood returning to the heart decreases, which must also decrease the volume leaving the heart.

Therefore the stroke volume diminishes. If the blood loss continues to a point where the heart rate has increased to 140 beats per minute to 'compensate', the stroke volume has decreased to 30 ml, then the cardiac output is down to 4200 ml per minute. The heart rate can no longer compensate for the blood loss and 'decompensation' occurs. However, the process of vasoconstriction, mentioned earlier, maintains some further compensatory ability.

5. Vasoconstriction

Decreased cardiac output stimulates a response from the brain to the smooth muscles in the walls of the small vessels. They contract, narrowing the lumen of the vessels (vasoconstriction). This process occurs in three stages:

- Those vessels that are over full and normally slightly dilated can be constricted a little without affecting tissue function (e.g., lungs, intestines, skeletal muscles). The extra blood improves venous return and in an adult there is a volume of about 500 ml. This stage is called *autotransfusion*.
- As stimulation from the brain continues, blood supply to all 'non vital structures' (i.e., other than brain and heart) is constricted. If we look at the skin, the most accessible of these non vital structures, we notice that it is pale, cold and clammy due to vasoconstriction of the peripheral vessels. Since the skin and other structures are receiving a reduced blood supply than is needed to maintain function, they are ischaemic and the result may be tissue damage.
- If the blood loss continues, the blood supply to 'life essential structures' (brain and heart is compromised. This is not due to vasoconstriction of their blood vessels, but rather the lack of circulating blood volume to maintain brain and heart function. This results in altered consciousness.

6. Limit of compensation

If blood loss continues, the body having reached the limit of response available through increased heart rate and vasoconstriction, can no longer maintain cardiac output and the blood pressure falls rapidly.

7. Decompensation

The sudden drop in blood pressure is the beginning of a critical sequence of events which, if not reversed rapidly, is fatal. The low blood pressure (hypotension) means that the blood supply to the tissues is inadequate. This ischaemia results in a decrease of oxygen and an increase in waste products in the cells. The brain, being the organ most sensitive to hypoxia, will fail, resulting in the patient collapsing. If the patient was upright and fell flat, this would provide temporary relief through the assistance of gravity improving venous return from the lower limbs. However, this is short-lived and with continued blood loss, ischaemic effects on the tissues leads to tissue damage. Coma and death then follow if the process is not stopped.

6

SUMMARY OF CLINICAL FEATURES OF SHOCK	
Appearance	Pale and cold
Breathing	Rapid and shallow
Heart rate	Rapid and becoming weak
Blood pressure	Decreasing
Conscious state	Decreasing

MANAGEMENT OF SHOCK

Early recognition and intervention is vital. Hypoxia is a significant problem and therefore high flow oxygen therapy is indicated. Treat the cause.

- **Control external blood loss**
- **Relieve the patient's pain**
- **Rest the heart.**

The problems of venous return and blood pressure can be reduced by posture. Earlier, mention was made of the effect of collapse providing a temporary reprieve. If we take this concept of 'autotransfusion' into mind and raise the lower limbs so that a head down position is achieved, the shock process may be slowed or minimised. Be careful not to overheat the patient as this will cause vasodilation of the peripheral vessels and compromise the body's compensatory processes. Maintain regular observation of the patient's physiological status and transport to the emergency department.

MEDICAL ANTI-SHOCK TROUSERS (MAST)

A valuable adjunct in the management of shock due to blood loss (hypovolaemia) is an inflatable garment which surrounds the lower limbs and torso. Medical anti-shock trousers (MAST) (Fig. 6.22) had their origins in the air force as a pressure suit for jet aircraft pilots, preventing blackout during high velocity flying manoeuvres, which created markedly changed gravitational forces. The concept was to pressurise the peripheral vascular fields to maintain an adequate circulatory capability, especially to the vital functional areas of the body.

In the emergency medical environment then, if a significant blood volume can be re-directed to the vital areas in incidents where severe blood loss has occurred, patient survival rates from trauma may be improved. The mechanism is believed to be one of raising peripheral vascular resistance rather than physically squeezing the blood from the

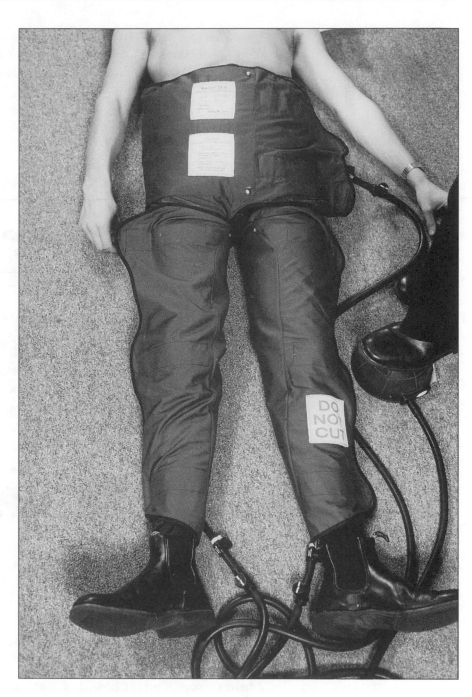

Fig. 6.22 A MAST suit prior to inflation. The suit is inflated one chamber at a time, beginning with the left leg. If the patient's breathing is impaired, slowly deflate the abdominal chamber.

lower limbs into the vital circulatory fields. However, regardless of the actual mechanism, the gain to circulation is of the order of 10 mmHg, which is significant in stabilising the hypovolaemic patient.

MAST is a useful garment in managing trauma to the lower limbs, providing pressure to control and splinting for fractures.

MAST should be used with caution in patients with trauma involving severe head injury, chest injury with suspected thoracic bleed, and pulmonary oedema.

TASK   Apply medical anti-shock trousers (MAST) to a patient   279

Once MAST is inflated, it is often much easier to cannulate and commence intravenous therapy, as the improvement in peripheral perfusion is to the extent that the veins of choice become more apparent.

On arrival at the emergency department, MAST should be left fully inflated until adequate intravenous volume replacement is running and ECG monitoring is commenced. This is the most potentially dangerous phase, as rapid deflation of the garment will have the effect of losing 2 units of blood in a matter of seconds, which can prove fatal to the patient.

> **IF YOU ARE UNFAMILIAR WITH MAST, DO NOT DEFLATE THE GARMENT**

MAST is always deflated sequentially, that is *one compartment at a time*. This may take up to 1 hour and at any stage, where the blood pressure falls rapidly by 5 mmHg or more, the suit should be re-inflated. Following a vital signs survey to confirm the patient's stability, the *torso compartment* is slowly deflated. Vital signs are then checked over a period of 10 minutes and if stable, *one leg compartment* can be deflated. Again, vital signs are monitored and the *other leg compartment* can be deflated if the patient is stable after the 10 minute check.

INTRAVENOUS THERAPY (IVT)

Resuscitation is the restoration of normal homeostasis. This is achieved by a variety of methods and procedures, one of which is the replacement and/or addition of fluids into the vascular field. The introduction of suitable fluids into the venous system is referred to as intravenous (IV) therapy or infusion.

There are TWO types of fluid, volume expanders and chemical replacements, used in the emergency environment.

Fluid to replace lost blood. Whole blood is the ideal replacement, but it is not available in pre-hospital management. Thus substitutes are widely used. The most common of these are Haemaccel and Stable Plasma Protein Solution (SPPS). Their action is to expand blood volume as a short term regime until whole blood can be infused in the emergency department.

Volume expanders are normally infused rapidly.

Fluid to replace chemicals. Fluid loss in burn injury, vomiting and diarrhoea results in salt loss. Solutions containing salt (normal saline or Hartmann's Solution) are usually infused over a relatively long period of time. Infusion is also used to keep a vein open and provide access for the introduction of other drugs when required. Commonly 5% dextrose (sugar in water) is used.

Chapter 9 (Advanced Life Support), provides more information on pharmacology and the commonly used intravenous drugs.

CANNULATION

Direct access to the circulatory system is achieved by the insertion of an indwelling catheter into a peripheral vein. The site for placement of the catheter will vary according to the patient's veins and clinical status. The most distal veins of the upper limbs are favoured but may be difficult to access if perfusion status is poor. The most common site used is the larger veins of the antecubital fossa. However, the cephalic veins of the fore-arm are an effective alternative site because the vein can be 'trapped' and immobilised with relative ease. The veins of the back of the hand are also a useful and stable site.

Before attempting cannulation, the patient's limb should be allowed to hang dependent for several minutes. This will help identify the vein of choice. Venous distension is further facilitated by applying a tourniquet above the elbow and stroking the vein in an upward direction.

'Trapping' or stabilising the vein is easier at a bifurcation, (division into branches) but if the site of choice is along a large vein, anchor the vein by applying traction to the skin around the vessel. The cephalic vein can be easily stabilised by adductive flexion of the wrist.

Avoid sites of *arterial pulsation* in close proximity and areas of injury. It is apreferable to avoid sites involving joints, although the antecubital fossa is a large vein site. If this is the site chosen, it is important to *immobilise the joint* to prevent dislodgement of the catheter.

Once the catheter is introduced into the vein and the IV line is attached, *remove the tourniquet*—a common cause of infusion cessation—and secure with tape to prevent movement. A generous loop of the IV line along the arm will provide added protection against dislodgement.

Check the infusion site for pain, swelling and discolouration periodically. These signs are evidence of venous rupture and infiltration of the tissues. If this occurs, apply direct pressure to the swelling and attempt cannulation at another site.

TASK   Insert a cannula into a peripheral vein   **280**

SETTING UP AN IV LINE

The solution to be infused (most commonly in a 'soft pack' but sometimes in glass flasks) has a protective cap seal to maintain the sterility of the contents. Care should be taken to keep it so.

Check the contents of the pack or flask to ensure that it is indeed the correct solution and that the expiry date has not been exceeded.

The infusion set consists of a large spike needle attached by a length of tubing to a drip chamber (some sets have an added filter unit). The drip chamber allows the flow rate to be counted accurately in drops per minute (dpm). A drip regulator is located on the length of tubing below the chamber and should be placed close to the chamber for ease of operation. The end of the tubing has a connector which is protected by a sterile cover. This cover should only be removed immediately prior to connecting the IV line to the indwelling catheter.

If a glass flask is in use, an airway needle is required to let air into the flask. This is always inserted first and again care must be taken to avoid contamination of the flask bung.

In the emergency setting, where volume expanders are in use, the drip rate is usually rapid (60-80 dpm). The slowest drip rate is about 20ml per hour. The standard adult IV set will deliver 15 drops per ml. Therefore, 20 ml per hour is a drip rate of 1 every 12 seconds (that is, 5 drops per minute).

The drips must be counted *accurately* and the prescribed rate maintained. If the fluid runs too fast, the drip must be slowed down, *but on no account stopped*, or a blockage of the catheter will occur.

The IV pack (or flask) must be secured either to an IV stand or a hook at a height of no less than 60 cm above the level of the patient's heart to maintain gravity feed. Ensure that the tubing is clear of obstructions and does not become kinked or pinched. Do not apply traction to the tubing as this may dislodge the cannula from the vein.

Trouble-shooting IV infusion

Problem	Action
1. Dislodgement of cannula	Turn off infusion. Re-insert cannula (if not trained, seek medical assistance).
2. Infusion ceases	Examine infusion site. • If it appears normal, turn infusion full on to flush clear. After successful flushing, reset drip rate. • If it appears abnormal, turn infusion off. Re-insert cannula (if not trained, leave off and seek medical assistance).
3. Air in infusion line	Encourage air to return up infusion line by: • holding the set slightly taut and flicking/tapping the line with a finger just below the air bubble. Then re-check the infusion rate; or, • turn infusion off and 'milk' the air up by wrapping the line around a pen. Then re-commence infusion. **Note:** This must be completed rapidly to prevent blockage of the cannula.
4. Empty pack/flask (no replacement)	Turn off infusion before the fluid level goes below the chamber.

THE PROBLEM OF HEART FAILURE

In Chapter 5 the problem of pulmonary oedema was raised as a respiratory emergency due to many causes. When the heart fails as an effective pump, blood backs up in the pulmonary or systemic circulatory fields, and sometimes in both. *Congestive cardiac failure* (CCF) is the term applied to this event of pulmonary oedema.

LEFT HEART FAILURE

Following AMI, which more commonly effects the left ventricle of the heart, the pumping efficiency of this chamber, providing the forward movement of blood to the body, is often seriously impaired. The right ventricle on the other hand is pumping with its normal efficiency. Therefore, blood backs up in the pulmonary circulation, the relatively short field between the heart and the lungs.

The effect is one of increasing pressure in the left atrium and pulmonary veins, which creates a hypostatic circulation in the pulmonary network. The engorgement of the pulmonary capillaries forces blood serum out of the capillaries into the alveoli. Because of the short circulatory field, pulmonary oedema manifests quite rapidly and is referred to as *acute left ventricular failure* following AMI. However, left heart failure may also be a chronic complication to valvular disorder, episodic myocardial ischaemia and cardiac dysrythmias.

The most significant clinical feature is severe dyspnoea, to the point where the patient is compelled to sit up to breathe. Breathing is noisy (often wheezy) and laboured and as the back log of blood increases, the neck veins become engorged. Cough often produces blood stained sputum.

RIGHT HEART FAILURE

Similarly, failure of the right ventricle, often following left heart failure, will cause back up of blood into the systemic circulation. This results in an increase of pressure in the peripheral veins, which causes fluid shift into surrounding tissues (oedema). Oedema is commonly seen in the lower limbs, in particular, the ankles.

The kidneys are unable to excrete the build up of fluids and salts from the body. Complicating the problem is the effect of the patient lying down to sleep. During the day, the fluid tends to remain in the extremities, but at rest, the fluid is reabsorbed and affects the lung fields. Therefore, during sleep, the patient develops a sudden onset dyspnoea, breathing being difficult unless sitting upright (orthopnoea). The patient may complain of abdominal pain, due to engorgement of the liver. This is the pattern of 'true' congestive cardiac failure.

MANAGEMENT

The first order management of heart failure is aimed at decreasing the oxygen demands and increasing alveolar oxygenation. High flow oxygen therapy and a sitting posture, preferably with the legs dependent is required. Maintain vital signs observations and transport to the emergency department. It is also helpful to the receiving medical officer if you can pass on a list of the patient's current medications.

A FEW WORDS ON TRAUMA

In Chapter 2, the problem of major external bleeding was discussed as part of the life threat management approach to an incident. Laceration of blood vessels is the most common traumatic insult to the cardiovascular system. But what if the damage involves a major vessel such as the aorta?

Aortic tear is not common, but indeed not rare. Severe blunt trauma to the trunk may result in damage to the arch of the aorta or along the descending path. Blood will leak into the layers of the vessel and track down the artery wall. This local dilation (aneurysm) may also be due to long-standing arteriosclerosis or hypertension. Pain is an intense 'tearing' sensation, felt across the chest wall, abdomen or lumbar region. The significant clinical feature is a pulsatile mass, usually palpable in the epigastrium.

The dilation of the vessel wall causes a drop in blood pressure, reducing the leakage. The risk comes when attempts to raise blood pressure commence. As the pressure increases, the tear may rupture, resulting in massive, uncontrolled bleeding, which is usually fatal.

As discussed in Chapter 2 in relation to the Vital Signs Survey, the potential for disaster of this nature can be identified if mechanism of the trauma and the physiological picture are combined. A patient who presents with extreme hypotension, with little or no external evidence of cause and who was involved in a high speed incident, is a potential victim of this type of injury. Early surgical intervention can save the patient and this incident is best managed by the 'load and go' method.

Severe blunt trauma to the thorax may also damage the myocardium, producing a similar clinical picture to that of AMI. However, if the myocardium is torn, there is the potential for blood loss into the pericardium. As blood fills the pericardial sac, stroke volume and cardiac output are compromised. The pulse becomes rapid and thready and the blood pressure falls, out of proportion to the blood loss. Neck veins become markedly distended as the circulatory field becomes engorged.

The accumulation of blood in the pericardium is referred to as *pericardial tamponade* and is a dire emergency. If not treated rapidly, cardiac arrest will occur. Again, this is a 'load and go' situation, maintaining high flow oxygen therapy en route to hospital. If cardiac arrest occurs, CPR should be commenced.

THE PROBLEM OF BURN INJURY

Thermal and chemical insult to the body will not only damage tissues, but also result in loss of body fluids (absolute fluid loss). While the immediate management of the burned victim involves pain relief and protection of the burn areas, the restoration of body fluid balance is of vital importance. This requires accurate assessment of the extent of the injury and urgent transport to the emergency department.

The majority of burn injuries occur in the home. Flame burns from open fires and barbecues are the most common, along with moist burns (scalds) from saucepans, pots, hot bath water and car radiators. Children and the elderly are the largest group of victims of moist burns.

ASSESSMENT

The assessment of burn injury is based on:

- The percentage of the body surface involved
- The depth of the burn injury
- The age and health status of the victim.

Area

The size of the area burned will determine the extent of body fluid loss. This assessment can be achieved by the use of the *Rule of Nines* (Fig. 6.23). In cases where the area of the injury is small, a useful measure is the area of the open hand of the victim. This is considered to be 1% of the body surface area. If the victim is an infant, the relative surfaces

6

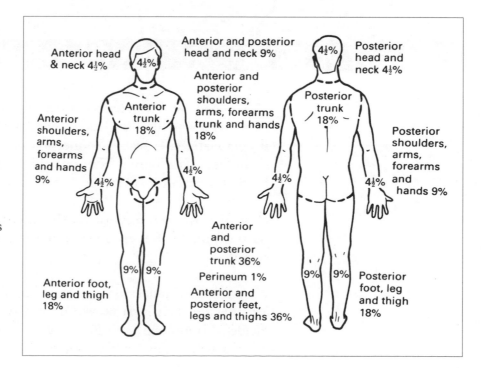

Fig. 6.23 The Rule of Nines is used for the assessment of the surface area of burns in adults. (Reproduced with permission from Chandler J 1991 Tabbner's nursing care: theory and practice, 2nd edition. Churchill Livingstone, Melbourne)

areas of the body are different from those of an adult and require a modified percentage scale (see Ch. 10).

An area of 15% or more in an adult is a serious burn. A burn area of greater than 10% is considered to be serious in a child. Smaller areas, especially those involving the face and hands, are serious burns regardless of their depth.

Depth

The depth of burn injuries is identified under 3 classifications:

- Superficial—burns involving the outer layers of the skin. (e.g., severe sunburn with blistering)
- Partial thickness (or deep dermal)—deeper burns in which most of the skin is destroyed, producing a mottled appearance and blistering
- Full thickness—destruction of the skin and underlying tissues, sometimes through to charring of the bone. The burned area appears white and charred.

The depth of the burn will influence the response to pain, depending on the extent of destruction of the pain fibres in the skin. Therefore, a superficial burn is likely to be more painful than a full thickness burn. In fact, victims with full thickness burns tend to have little pain response.

Age and health status

Age and general health status should also be considered in the assessment. The very young and the elderly do not tolerate significant fluid loss and if the victim is in poor health at the time of the injury, the additional loss of homeostasis will overwhelm normal compensatory mechanisms.

MANAGEMENT OF BURN INJURY

The immediate care of burn injuries requires cooling of the area. This helps to prevent further tissue damage and often helps to relieve pain. If cold water is available, immersion of a localised burn should be performed. If the burn is extensive, the application of cold compresses for 5-10 minutes is advisable.

Never immerse a patient totally in cold water or treat burns with ice packs. Severe hypothermia and death of tissue may result.

In most circumstances of flame burns, the ambulance crew arrives well after the initial crisis. However, if the patient is alight on arrival at the incident, smothering the flames with a blanket is an alternative if dousing with water is not an option. Smouldering clothing will cause further injury and should be quickly removed. Cut clothing off if necessary. Clothing that has adhered to the body should be left until arrival at the emergency department.

> **NEVER TAKE OFF BURNING OR SMOULDERING CLOTHING OVER THE HEAD. THIS MAY CAUSE SERIOUS DISFIGUREMENT TO THE FACE**

Analgesia is required for superficial burns. However, as mentioned earlier, full thickness burns tend not to be very painful and often pain relief is not required.

The burned area should be covered with burn dressings or clean linen to minimise micro-organism contamination. The problem of infection is often a critical factor in the recovery of the patient.

Intravenous therapy should be commenced as soon as possible. If this can be commenced in the field, Hartmann's Solution or normal saline should be used. The rate per hour is calculated by:

$$\frac{\% \text{ of burn x body weight}}{5}$$

Airway burns

Burn injuries to the upper torso, neck and face may involve damage to the respiratory tract. The inhalation of hot gases may damage the mucous membranes, resulting in oedema of the airway, causing obstruction. The airway is the first priority in cases of burn injury patients with damage to lips, singed facial hair and especially if they present with a harsh cough or stridor. Oxygen therapy is an essential element of management and if it is not possible to apply a face mask because of facial injury, a field of oxygen can be provided by holding the mask close to the patient's face. The oxygen flow rate should be 8–10 litres per minute to maintain an effective concentration of oxygen in the field.

Electrical burns

Electrical burns may be more serious than they first appear and are often accompanied by respiratory or cardiac arrest.

> **IF STILL IN CONTACT, DO NOT TOUCH THE PATIENT UNTIL THE ELECTRICAL SOURCE IS DISCONNECTED**

If the ambulance crew must remove the patient from the source, extreme care must be taken and under no circumstances should an attempt be made to remove a patient from high voltage sources. Low voltage sources may be managed by the use of insulating materials, such as a *dry* wooden stick (a long wooden splint is ideal) or wad of newspaper.

The management of electrical burns is limited to resuscitation (CPR) if required and covering the entrance and exit burn sites. Tissue damage is mostly internal—along the path through which the current passed—and requires surgical management in the hospital environment. If the patient is conscious, analgesia may be required and oxygen therapy should be administered in-transit. Transport to the emergency department should be without delay.

Chemical burns

Chemicals, commonly acids and strong alkalis, are frequent causes of burn injuries in industry. However, caustic materials, in the form of household cleaning agents, are responsible for many burn incidents among children.

Rapid removal and neutralisation of the chemical is the immediate priority. Copious amounts of running water should be used to wash the material from the body and should be continued until all traces of the chemical have been flushed from the skin. Clothing and jewelry must be removed to ensure that no further burning occurs from chemicals soaked into clothes or trapped beneath the jewelry.

DO NOT USE WATER WITH DRY POWDER CHEMICALS

Dry powder chemicals may react with water, increasing tissue damage. Brush the powder from the skin.

Chemical burns to the eye from splashes are best treated by holding the eye, with the eyelid open, under gentle running water for at least 15 minutes. An eye irrigation set is useful to continue the flushing during transport to the emergency department and should be continued until specialist medical assistance is available.

CASE HISTORY

You and your partner have just cleared the emergency department of the local hospital and are returning to the station on a bright, sunny spring afternoon. The despatcher calls via radio:

> *Proceed to 33 Howard Avenue, Oxley Heights, a male patient complaining of chest pain. Case number 190 at 1452 hours.*

Response time is 6 minutes and on arrival, a middle aged women directs you to the livingroom where you find her 63 year old husband reclining on the lounge, pale and sweaty and in obvious distress.

1. **What is the approach to differentiating chest pain?**

2. **Describe the pain assessment process.**

The physiological assessment reveals:

- *Heart rate 130 weak and irregular*
- *Respiratory rate 18 laboured*
- *Blood pressure 95 systolic*
- *Capillary refill >2 seconds.*

3. **What is your initial treatment?**

The cardiac monitor is attached to the patient and you prepare to move the patient. The ECG trace recorded initially is:

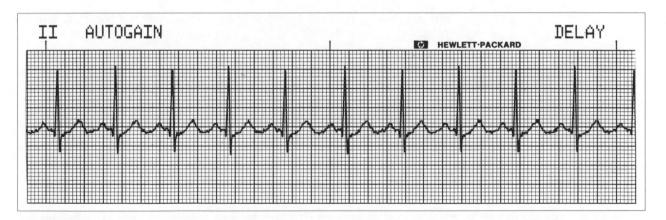

4. **What is the name of the rhythm in the ECG strip above?**

You establish that the patient has a past history of AMI and is currently prescribed Digoxin 0.25 mg, Frusemide 40 mg and Slow K. You and your partner are about to lift the patient on to the stretcher, when he gasps and collapses into unconsciousness. The vital signs are now:

- *Heart rate nil*
- *Respiratory rate nil*
- *Non-responsive to stimuli.*

ECG shows:

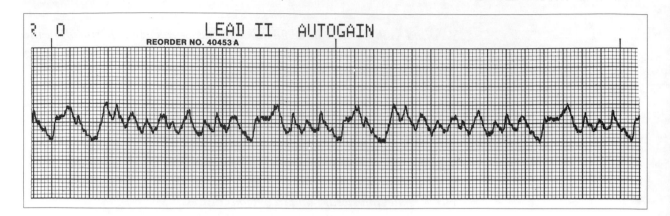

5. **What is the ECG rhythm?**

6. **What action do you take?**

The attempt to defibrillate is unsuccessful and you continue CPR for 2 minutes before a further defibrillation attempt.

7. **What is the ratio of compressions to ventilations for 2 rescuer CPR?**

After 2 minutes of CPR the check for heart rate and rhythm shows nil output and ventricular fibrillation.

8. **What further action do you take?**

The outcome of the second defibrillation is successful and the ECG is now displaying

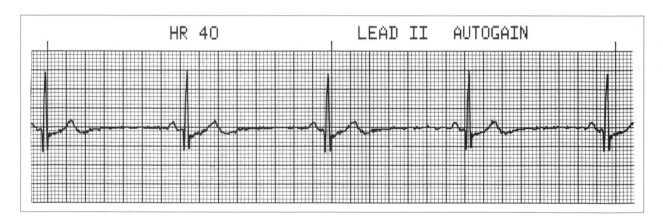

You palpate the pulse and confirm a weak output at a rate of 50 per minute. Respirations are still absent.

9. **What is your next action?**

10. **Using your patient care record, complete the documentation for the case.**

(Answers on page 302)

FURTHER READING

Alpert & Francis 1987 Manual of coronary care. Little Brown, Boston

Anon1984 Cardiovascular disorders. Springhouse Corporation Springhouse,

Hampton J R 1986 The ECG in practice. Churchill Livingstone, Edinburgh

Smith B 1984 Heart attack and back. Reed, Sydney

6

CHAPTER 7
Of conscious status

The nervous system and disorders of altered consciousness are an area of study which tends to be glossed over, because of its complexity. A commonsense approach in this chapter to the structure and function of the central nervous system and the essentials of assessing altered consciousness, provides a practical perspective to problem management.

Head injury, metabolic disorder, poisons and drugs are incorporated under conscious status, as the primary effects relate to nervous impairment.

Topics covered

CNS at a glance
Conscious status assessment
Head and spinal injuries
Non-traumatic coma
Poisons and drugs

All activities and functions within the body occur under the surveillance and control of the central nervous system. Changes in homeostasis are acted upon immediately by stimulating the actions of the various organs and support mechanisms to restore balance. Every movement we execute is a controlled purposeful act, requiring many separate functions to be coordinated to bring about the act. Consider the facts that we breathe continually at a rate suitable to our oxygen requirements, our heart rate increases and decreases according to our physical efforts, and a host of other automatic functions occur of which we remain very much unaware.

Such actions require a highly sophisticated computer with linkages to every part of the body. The human brain is that 'computer' and the spinal cord and peripheral nerves are the linkages. Any disturbance to the brain or damage to the neurological wiring, will result in dysfunction of part or parts of the body. If the brain is insulted, our conscious awareness is impaired.

The most common and significant insult to the brain is *hypoxia* and therefore the *vital* elements of patient care must be *good airway maintenance and adequate oxygenation*.

CNS AT A GLANCE

Aim

To develop an understanding of the nervous system

Learning plan

1. Read the text information
2. Supplement reading with a more comprehensive anatomy and physiology text
3. Check your understanding using the knowledge check

BRAIN

The brain is housed within and protected by the skull. Further protection is afforded by the soft tissue coverings (meninges) and a fluid barrier (cerebrospinal fluid). However, it becomes apparent that this protection is somewhat limited if you consider the effect of pressure following injury to the brain. Unlike most other tissues in the body, which have room to swell, the skull vault provides the brain with very little space. Brain tissue cannot withstand pressure and dysfunction is the result. If you further consider that the brain, within the skull vault, has a massive circulatory field supplying oxygen and vital nutrients, it is obvious that the effect of brain swelling will be to severely impede blood flow. The outcome is an hypoxic spiral, which exacerbates cerebral dysfunction. For this reason, airway maintenance and oxygen therapy are the essentials of head injury management.

The brain is one of the largest organs of the body (Fig. 7.1). It makes up only about 2% of total body weight, yet uses some 20% of the oxygen utilised within the body. The 4 principal sections of the brain are the cerebrum, diencephalon, brainstem and cerebellum.

The cerebrum constitutes the bulk of the brain, in which all conscious functions (e.g., seeing, speaking and moving) are controlled. It is also the area responsible for higher functions (thought and reasoning).

The diencephalon comprises the *thalamus* and *hypothalamus*, surrounded by the cerebrum (Fig. 7.2). The principal functions relate to sensory interpretation (pain, temperature, pressure) and control of most homeostatic mechanisms. The hypothalamus is also the centre associated with strong emotions (rage and aggression).

The brainstem is found at the base of the brain, and contains the 'primitive' functionary centres critical to survival (respiration and circulation). The principal motor and sensory centres for heart and lung function are housed in the *medulla*, the inferior portion of the brainstem, continuous with the spinal cord. It is also the point in the

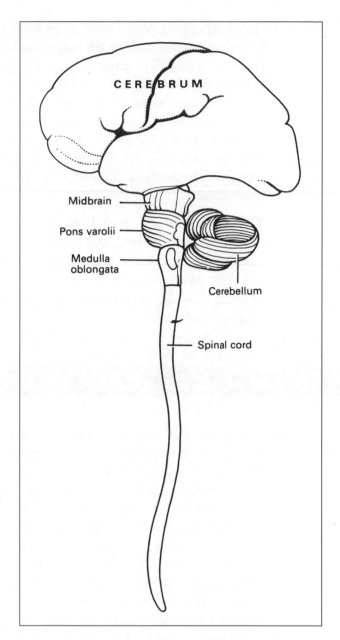

Midbrain

Pons varolii

Medulla
oblongata

Cerebellum

Spinal cord

Fig. 7.1 The central nervous system consists of the various parts of the brain and the spinal cord.
(Reproduced with permission from Wilson K J W 1990 Ross & Wilson: Anatomy and physiology in health and illness, 7th edition. Churchill Livingstone, Edinburgh)

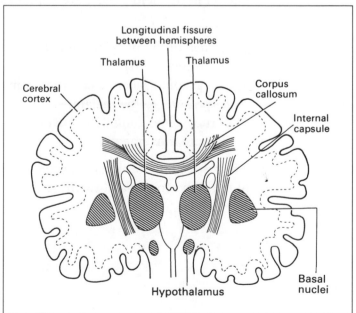

Fig. 7.2 A section of the cerebrum showing the location of the two principal components of the diencephalon and some connecting nerve fibres.
(Reproduced with permission from Wilson K J W 1990 Ross & Wilson: Anatomy and physiology in health and illness, 7th edition. Churchill Livingstone, Edinburgh)

circuit where the 'cross-over' of pathways (decussation) occurs. The resultant effect is that the left side of the body is controlled by the right cerebral hemisphere and the right side by the left hemisphere. The value of this decussation phenomenon is unknown.

The *reticular formation* of the medulla is also a noteworthy structure, maintaining conscious levels and responsible for arousal. If you are struck on the mandible (lower jaw), the impact distorts the brainstem sending a rapid series of impulses to the cerebrum. This volley of impulses overwhelms the reticular cells and results in loss of consciousness.

The cerebellum is located adjacent to the brainstem and inferior to the cerebrum. The principal functions relate to maintaining balance, equilibrium and the coordination of movements. Injury to this area, although rare, results in loss of coordination and balance. It is also thought that the cerebellum may play a part in emotions such as pleasure and anger.

SPINAL CORD

The spinal cord is the second of the major structures comprising the central nervous system. It commences as the continuation of the medulla and extends down the spinal column to the level of the 2nd lumbar vertebra, a length of about 43 cm in an adult.

Like the brain, the cord is protected by the meninges and cerebrospinal fluid. The bony canal, formed by the projections of each vertebra provides more firm protection.

The principal function of the spinal cord is to convey *sensory* information from the organs and periphery to the brain (ascending tracts) and *motor* impulses from the brain to the body (descending tracts). From the practical viewpoint—managing the spinal injury patient in the field—there are 3 important tracts:

- posterior columns—which provide an awareness of the exact *position* of the body and the direction of their movement (proprioception)
- lateral spinothalamic column—conveys senses of *pain* and *temperature* to the thalamus
- corticospinal column—conveys motor impulses for precise and discrete movements.

The assessment for spinal injury should therefore include observations of position sense, pain, temperature and movement.

AUTONOMIC NERVOUS SYSTEM

At the beginning of this chapter, reference was made to the many body functions that occur automatically and continuously in the maintenance of homeostasis. These functions involve excitation of some areas to increase activity and inhibition of others to decrease activity. The autonomic nervous system, a 'system within a system', is responsible for the coordination of these subconscious functions. The system consists of 2 parts:

- The sympathetic or excitory part, is concerned with expending energy
- The parasympathetic or inhibitory part, which essentially decreases activities, restoring and conserving energy.

Disturbances to homeostasis, whether due to physical insult or emotion (e.g., stress and fear), activate the sympathetic part, causing a series of physiological responses. Collectively, these responses are referred to as the 'fight-or-flight' response, the necessary preparations to take appropriate action. For example, consider the requirements of the body to act:

Cells will need a good oxygen supply.	=	Respiratory bronchioles dilate and breathing rate increases.
Cells will need more glucose to create energy.	=	Liver glycogen is converted to glucose to increase blood sugar levels.
A good transport system is needed to supply cells.	=	Heart rate increases and blood vessels to muscles and essential organs dilate.

Non essential processes to this action, such as the functions of digestion, are slowed or even ceased. Consider further, the compensatory actions of the body in the shock process. Sympathetic stimulations increase heart rate to maintain cardiac output; vasoconstriction maintains effective blood pressure levels. Parasympathetic stimulations tend to slow down body functions and in many instances have a directly opposite effect from that of sympathetic stimulations (e.g., decelerating influence on the sinoatrial node in the heart, decreasing heart rate and the force of contraction.) However, it is parasympathetic stimulation which activates the digestive processes and genitourinary system functions.

Thus, the autonomic nervous system plays an important role in stabilising the normal physiological states of the body.

KNOWLEDGE CHECK

The brain

1. Apart from the skull, what other protection is afforded to the brain?

2. What are the 4 principal sections of the brain and their functions?

3. What are the 2 components of the diencephalon?

4. In which section of the brain is the medulla located and what are its main functions?

The spinal cord

5. Describe the position of the spinal cord

6. What are the names of the 3 important spinal cord tracts and their prime functions?

Turn to page 303 to check your answers.

CONSCIOUS STATUS ASSESSMENT

Aim

To develop an objective approach to assessing altered consciousness

Learning plan

1. Read the text information
2. Practise the 3 sections of observations
3. Check your understanding using the knowledge check

In the primary survey, the concern was simply whether the patient responded to 'shout and shake'. When gathering vital signs information to provide a full picture of the patient's physiological status, a more detailed and concise observation of conscious status is necessary.

For many years, terms such as confused, stuporous, semi-comatose and comatose were used to describe altered conscious states. Such words were difficult to interpret and somewhat meaningless as a measure of status.

In the early 1970s at the University of Glasgow, Teasdale and Jennett developed the first quantitative and repeatable coma scale. The *Glasgow Coma Scale* (GCS) has become the universal standard for describing and recording conscious status. Rather than confining the assessment to a single, subjective word, the GCS provides an objective appraisal divided into three sections (Fig. 7.3). Given that *standard stimuli* are used, this system of observation is sensitive to deterioration in conscious status.

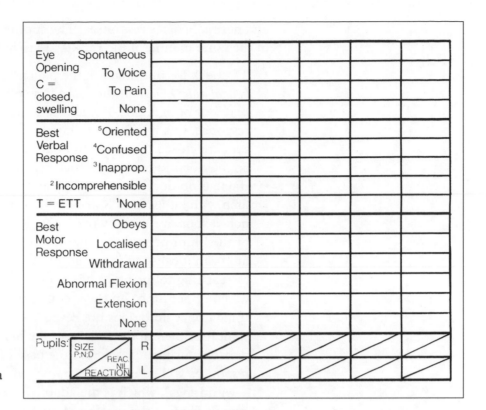

Fig. 7.3 The Glasgow Coma Scale.

Eye opening as seen in Figure 7.3, there are four responses. Only one response is charted:

- If the patient is conscious and opening his or her eyes spontaneously, place a cross on the top line
- If the patient's eyes are closed, use a verbal stimulus (e.g., the patient's name). This is a second line response
- If there is no response to verbal stimulus, a pain stimulus is necessary. The safest method is to press the *blunt end of a pen* onto the mid-sternum. If the eyes open to the pain stimulus, a third line response is recorded
- If there is no response to the pain stimulus, a bottom line response is charted.

Best verbal response is divided into five responses and as the title suggests, record only the best response observed. A suitable stimulus is to ask 'Do you know where you are?'

- If the response is correct, an oriented result is recorded
- If the response is incorrect, record a second line response—confused
- If the patient answers with something totally irrelevant (or 'Anglo-saxon') an inappropriate result is recorded
- If moans, groans and unintelligible sounds are elicited, record a fourth line response of incomprehensible
- Failure to respond is recorded as a bottom line response.

Best motor response focuses on movement and is aimed at determining neurological function or dysfunction, not specifically evidence of spinal or limb injury. This is the most complex section of the scale and normally of six responses. The stimuli must always be performed in the same manner if the results are to have any meaning.

- To check for obeying, ask the patient: '*Squeeze my fingers with both of your hands*' at the same time offering the *index and middle fingers* of both hands. Avoid any action which might elicit a grasp response, this is difficult to interpret. However, if the patient's eyes are closed (e.g., due to injury), you may touch the patient on the dorsum of the first metacarpal.
- If one limb does not respond, chart the action of the responding limb with either L or R as obeys and proceed to persecute the non-responsive limb by pain stimulus. This is attempted firstly by the blunt pen on mid-sternum method to assess whether the limb can localise to the point of the pain. If the patient responds by reaching to the point of stimulus, chart L or R (depending on which upper limb) on the second line for localises.
- If the upper limb does not respond to localising pain, take the stimulus down to the fingers of the hand and apply nailbed pressure, using a pen across the base of thumb nail. One of four responses will be elicited:
  —withdrawal, which is the adaptive flexor response to noxious stimuli. This is the making of angles in the limb (at elbow and wrist, and even the fingers)
  —flexion, which is an abnormal twisting of the limb away from the stimulus
  —extension, which is a straightening of the limb, often with a twisting of the wrist and fingers, again a maladaptive response
  —no response, which is charted on the bottom line of the motor response section.

A single set of GCS observations is of little significance, but a series of assessments over a short period of time will provide a picture of the trend in neurological function.

In the old charting systems *pupillary response* was the only sign of significance, although often too late if the problem was an intracranial bleed. If the GCS is used properly, repeated with the same stimulus methods, deterioration will be evident long before significant pupil changes occur. Size and pupil reactivity is not therefore as important, but it is still useful to include in the data collection. Pupil size is charted according to a scale of 8 diameters or as shown in Figure 7.3, simply either pin-point (P), normal (N) or dilated (D).

The Glasgow Coma Scale is scored with a numeric value highest for the top line responses (e.g., 5 for an oriented verbal response, or 6 for obeys with motor response) and decreasing to 1 for a nil response in each section. However, as with other scoring systems, its value is really only in a statistical sense because a pitfall exists in interpreting a single number comprising 3 variables. For example, is it a case of the patient having a good motor response but a poor verbal one? Or is the patient completely oriented, but cannot move? What is of more significance to the emergency department is a statement of the 3 variables. The most *vital element* of a conscious status assessment is whether the *observations* taken are *changing* and whether the clinical picture is *improving or deteriorating.*

KNOWLEDGE CHECK

7. What are the 3 variables of the Glasgow Coma Scale?

8. List the responses for each of the 3 variables of the Glasgow Coma Scale.

9. What is the significance of GCS over other conscious status assessment approaches?

Turn to page 303 to check your answers.

HEAD AND SPINAL INJURIES

Aim

To develop an understanding of the problems of head and spinal injury and develop skills in their management

Learning plan

1. Read the text information
2. Check your understanding using the knowledge check
3. Practise the assessment and management of patients presenting with traumatic coma

7

THE PROBLEM OF HEAD INJURY

Head injury is one of the most significant causes of death and critical trauma in traffic crashes. Intracranial injury results from rapid deceleration of the brain following impact with the rigid skull vault. The compression of the delicate brain mass leads to shearing and tearing, resulting in laceration or contusion with subsequent haemorrhage. Loss of the normal regulatory mechanisms controlling cerebral blood supply causes engorgement of cerebral blood vessels, which compromises venous drainage and results in a rise in intracranial pressure.

Rising intracranial pressure will cause changes to other vital signs. Normally you expect bleeding to cause the compensatory actions of an increase in pulse rate and respirations and, later, a fall in blood pressure. The clinical picture of increasing intracranial pressure has 2 elements. There is a slow, abnormal respiratory pattern initially (but as the pressure continues, breathing becomes rapid and sudden respiratory arrest may occur). The second element is a slowing pulse rate accompanied by a rising blood pressure.

The pre-hospital care of head-injured patients requires attention to five critical tasks:

- Precise and detailed conscious status assessment (GCS)
- Frequent total physiological status surveys
- Details of the mechanism of injury, e.g,.where the patient was in the incident, what force or impact was involved, what happened to the patient (thrown out of the vehicle, restrained by a seat-belt)
- Good airway maintenance—*a vital factor*
- High flow oxygen, with assisted ventilation if necessary.

A patient who has sustained significant trauma to the head may have a cervical spine injury. Head injured patients should be treated as cervical injuries until proven otherwise.

Skull fracture

There are 6 types of bone injury to the skull.

Linear fractures are breaks in the continuity of the bone, but without alteration in the relationship of the bone parts. They are usually only evident from X-ray examination and are normally of little clinical significance.

Blows between the orbits may shatter the ethmoid sinuses and the roof of the nose. Blows higher up on the forehead may cause fractures, which cross the frontal sinus. Frontal fractures may produce discharge of cerebrospinal fluid (CSF) and even brain tissue from the nose.

Fractures of the orbit, including the zygoma, may restrict eye movement and result in 'double vision', with bruising limited to the orbital tissue. There may be subconjunctival bruising and blindness of one eye if the fracture involves the optic foramen.

Depressed fractures range from simple buckling in the skull (pond fracture), following a blow from a blunt object, to comminuted ('gutter' fracture) from a high velocity blow. The inner table of the skull may be fragmented, causing meningeal and brain tissue damage.

Base of skull fractures usually declare themselves by bleeding (often watery blood, mixed with CSF) from the ear canal and nose. This bleeding may come from nothing more serious than an injury of the ear or nose, but the escape of watery blood or blood stained watery liquid leaves no doubt that the meningeal barrier is torn.

Jaw fractures, both maxilla and mandible and dislocation of the mandible, may result from direct blunt trauma. The significant complication is airway impairment from soft tissue damage, bleeding, and broken or dislodged teeth.

Management

There is little that can be done to manage skull fractures, with the exception of covering open fracture sites and controlling bleeding. Most fractures in this region tend to be supported by the adjacent bony structures. However, in the case of base of skull fracture, the patient should be placed in a side posture; the ear, from which fluid discharge is draining, facing down. This will allow further drainage of fluid to prevent retention within the skull vault. A dressing should be placed over the ear to reduce the potential for infection, given that there is now an open communication to the meningeal region.

Mandibular fractures require support, but avoid firm bandaging, as this may compromise the airway. Transport the patient in a side posture to assist drainage.

THE PROBLEM OF SPINAL INJURY

Trauma to the spine and spinal cord is a catastrophic event. The effects are not only disastrous for the victim, but pose long term difficulties for the family. The outcome of spinal trauma frequently depends upon the immediate management of the victim at the scene. A thorough pre-hospital assessment and appropriate care may mean the difference between permanent disability and minor neurological deficit.

Injury to the vertebral column, spinal cord, or both, may result from trauma to the head and neck, shoulders and back. The type and degree of force exerted on the spinal column will determine the extent of initial damage. Instability of the ligaments supporting the spine may lead to further injury if the management and movement of the victim is inadequate. The most common sites of injury are the cervical vertebral region (C5 and C6) and the middle region—thoracic and lumbar (T12 and L1). These sites usually result in the greatest degree of spinal cord injury and are frequently seen in motor car crashes where sudden rotation and hyperflexion occurs.

Hyperextension injuries, from falls or crashes, most commonly affect C4 and C5 and are usually seen in older victims with bony degeneration of the vertebrae. The cause of injury in the elderly patient is often quite trivial in nature. Compression injury to the spinal column, occurring in falls from significant height and diving accidents, tend to be more stable. This relative stability is due to the vertebrae and ligaments frequently remaining intact and therefore the extent of damage is sometimes less serious. The common sites of compression are C5–C6 and T12–L1.

7

Assessment

The assessment of the patient in suspected spinal injury involves considering the history of the incident and completing a physical examination of both motor and sensory functions. The mechanism of injury, discussed in Chapter 2, will help in determining the probability of spinal trauma. If the patient is unconscious, this information becomes vital.

Any unconscious patient involved in an accident and sustaining injury to the face and head, should be treated as a spinal injury victim until proven otherwise.

The conscious patient may provide information about the accident and what happened, as well as evidence of sensations and inability to move limbs. However, it is not uncommon for patients not to realise that they are paralysed, because of the pain associated with injuries.

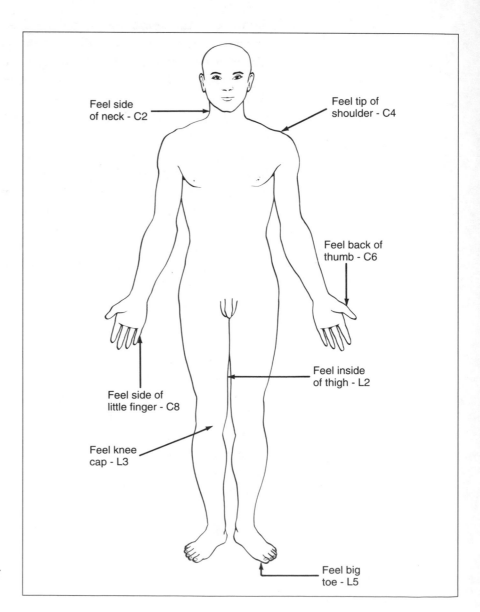

Fig. 7.4 The sensory survey points for locating the site of possible spinal injury.

Feel side of neck - C2

Feel tip of shoulder - C4

Feel back of thumb - C6

Feel inside of thigh - L2

Feel side of little finger - C8

Feel knee cap - L3

Feel big toe - L5

The physical examination must survey both motor and sensory functions. There may be motor damage (loss of movement) without sensory loss or vice versa. The level at which sensory loss is found and/ or motor deficit is noted, indicates the site of injury.

Sensory survey

The assessment requires responses to *light touch* and *pain*. The forehead, unless severely injured, usually has normal sensory responses and can be used as a guide to establishing the patient's normal response level. The assessment should take only about 1 minute and focuses on finding where sensation changes. An understanding of the spinal innervation (Fig. 7.4) then can be applied to locate the site of injury. Sensory check of the thorax (T4) is performed at the *mid-axillary lines*, not mid-clavicular, because the cervical branches (C2, C3 and C4) also provide sensory communication to the nipple line.

Motor survey

Upper and lower limbs are assessed by asking the patient to perform a range of movements.

Upper limbs

Action	Nerve origin
Shrug the shoulders	C5
Bend the elbow	C5
Push the wrist back	C6
Make a fist	C8

Lower limbs

Action	Nerve origin
Flex the hip	L1 and L2
Extend the knee	L3
Bend the ankle up	L4
Push the foot down	L5 and S1

Motor assessment of the thorax and abdomen is performed by observing the activity of the intercostal and abdominal muscles.

The unconscious trauma patient. An assessment for spinal injury in the trauma patient who is unconscious should be conducted, especially if there is evidence of facial or head injury. If the forces exerted on the head were enough to cause altered consciousness, then there is likely to be damage to the cervical spine, often resulting in quadriplegia.

Observe the patient's respiratory movements. Note if the pattern is 'paradoxical' (i.e., the abdomen rises on inspiration and falls on exhalation, with no chest movement). This means that the patient is breathing diaphragm dependent and innervation to the intercostal muscles is lost.

Check for response to pain stimulus. Loss of pain response occurs only when the patient is deeply unconscious. If there is a response to pain stimulus, it will help in locating the level of injury. For example, if nail bed pressure applied to the thumb and fingers results in a response, but when applied to the toes fails to cause response, there is evidence to suggest paraplegia.

Blood pressure can provide further suspicion of possible spinal cord damage. If the patient has a pulse within normal limits or a bradycardia, but is hypotensive (systolic pressure <100 mmHg), a spinal lesion exists until proven otherwise.

Spinal injury causes circulatory dilatation due to loss of sympathetic nervous control. Male patients with suspected spinal injury will have an erect penis (priapism), due to dilatation of the vessels of the penis.

Management

The management of the spinally injured patient, as is true of all patients, requires firstly attending to life threatening problems—airway, breathing and circulatory problems. If these critical problems are present, they must take priority over the spinal injury. However, care must be taken during airway management to not produce a vagal stimulus. Following cord injury, the parasympathetic branch of the nervous system may be intact and unopposed. The use of suction or the insertion of an oropharyngeal airway may cause an unopposed vagal stimulus which may lead to cardiac arrest.

Use suction and insert oropharyngeal airways with care to reduce vagal stimulus.

Of vital importance is the effect of hypoxia on the injured spinal cord. Underperfusion of the cord—due to the compensatory mechanisms of the shock process—will result in further damage. Ventilatory function is impeded, due to impairment of the chest wall and abdominal muscles, resulting in diaphragm dependent breathing. Therefore high flow oxygen support, and where necessary assisted ventilation with bag and mask, are important elements of the management strategy.

The movement of the patient should be performed with regard to the spinal injury.

Move the patient in one piece, without rotating or twisting.

Immobilisation of the spine is vital before lifting or moving the patient. The cervical spine is the least supported region and requires the application of a cervical collar. Where possible, lift the patient in the position found and avoid multiple movements. The use of lifting devices, e.g., Jordon Frame or a blanket, will minimise the tendency to rotate or twist the patient. Full spine immobilisation devices, e.g., the Kendrik Extrication Device (KED), provide a safe method of handling the patient.

Extrication of the spinally injured patient from a motor vehicle should involve a 'team' lift and must not be rushed. Think about the best exit route from the car before commencing—the shortest route may not be the best route. Bucket seats can be reclined, making the rear door a suitable and wider exit point, clear of obstructions in the front of the passenger compartment.

Transport to the emergency department should be without delay, but a smooth ride is required. This does not mean that it is necessary to travel slowly. Normal speed may be used, but avoid sharp cornering, heavy acceleration and braking.

KNOWLEDGE CHECK

10. What are the 4 critical tasks in the management of the head injured patient?

11. What are the common sites where spinal injury occurs?

12. Describe the 2 sections of the physical survey for spinal injury.

13. What are the critical factors in the management of the spine injured patient?

Turn to page 303 to check your answers.

NON-TRAUMATIC COMA

Aim

To develop an understanding of the causes of non-traumatic coma and their management

Learning plan

1. Read the text information
2. Check your understanding using the knowledge check
3. Practise the assessment and management of patients presenting with non-traumatic coma.

The cells of the brain are totally dependent on a continuous supply of blood. Any interference to this blood supply, even for short periods, will cause dysfunction and cellular death may result.

7

CEREBROVASCULAR ACCIDENT (CVA)

The cause of interference to cerebral blood flow frequently encountered in the pre-hospital environment is the CVA, or 'stroke'. Cerebral thrombosis in elderly people, as a result of arteriosclerosis of a cerebral artery is a common cause. Haemorrhage into the brain, due to rupture of a cerebral artery as a result of hypertension may produce a CVA in younger age groups. A third cause is a cerebral embolus, a moving or detached clot (air or fat globule), which lodges in a cerebral artery. This is often seen in patients with heart disease and may occur in victims of multiple trauma, chest injury or long bone fracture.

The result will depend on the location and extent of tissue death. Transient ischaemic attacks (TIA), a series of 'small strokes' of short duration (usually up to 10 minutes), are experienced by some patients prior to a major CVA. TIA is evidenced by short term speech disorder, weakness (hemiparesis) or paralysis of one side of the body. Between episodes, the neurologic clinical picture is normal.

CVA is usually rapid in onset and characterised by:

- Numbness or paralysis of the extremities, affecting one side of the body (hemiplegia)
- Headache and confusion, sometimes with inappropriate behaviour (excessive crying or laughing)
- Difficulty in speaking (dysphasia), often with slurred speech of which the patient is unaware.

Altered consciousness, loss of bladder and bowel control may occur and some patients will convulse.

Management

A CVA is a terrifying experience for the conscious patient, so *good communication* and *reassurance* are essentials of management. If the patient cannot speak, *do not assume that he or she cannot understand.* Understanding can be tested during conscious status assessment, by the simple command 'Squeeze my fingers'.

Protect paralysed limbs from damage and position the patient comfortably (usually recumbent). If the patient is unconscious, place in a stable side posture. Administer oxygen via a face mask and transport to the emergency department safely and steadily.

DIABETIC EMERGENCIES

The brain depends entirely on the constant supply of oxygen and glucose transported by the blood. If the blood sugar level changes markedly, brain tissue is compromised. Diabetes mellitus is a disorder of carbohydrate metabolism, due to a deficiency in the secretion of insulin from the pancreas or the diminished effectiveness of insulin, which causes disturbance to normal blood sugar levels.

If blood sugar levels are too low or too high the delicate balance of glucose regulation is upset and may lead to a life threatening emergency.

Hypoglycaemia (low blood sugar) is a life threatening emergency, requiring urgent replacement of glucose.

- **History**
  —too much insulin
  —no food
  —unusually vigourous exercise
- **Onset**
  —rapid, normally in 'good health' just before
- **Clinically**
  —pale, cold, clammy skin
  —full (bounding) pulse, normal or raised blood pressure
  —normal or shallow breathing
  —excited and often aggressive followed by rapid loss of consciousness, tremor and convulsions may occur.

If the patient is conscious, give oral glucose and commence high flow oxygen therapy. The patient should be transported to the emergency department for further assessment and stabilisation.

If the patient is unconscious, airway maintenance, oxygen therapy and rapid IV glucose infusion is required. If IV is available, give 50% dextrose IV or IVI, depending on your service's protocol.

If IV is not available, maintain the patient's airway, give high flow oxygen and transport rapidly to the emergency department.

Hyperglycaemia or diabetic ketoacidosis (high blood sugar level) is not life threatening, but the patient may be at risk due to airway obstruction if unconscious.

- **History**
  —omission or too little insulin
  —dietary indiscretion
  —infection or digestive disturbance
- **Onset**
  —usually slow with ill health several days before
- **Clinically**
  —flushed, dry, hot skin
  —weak, rapid pulse with a low blood pressure
  —laboured breathing (air hunger) with a 'fruity' odour on the breath
  —abdominal pain, nausea and vomiting
  —excessive thirst
  —excessive urine output
  —may be 'drowsy', sometimes unconscious

7

Treatment for hyperglycaemia is limited to oxygen therapy and transport to the emergency department for stabilisation. If the patient is unconscious, maintain airway care and transport in a stable side position.

EPILEPSY

Epileptic seizures can be described as a brief disorder of cerebral function, usually associated with altered consciousness and accompanied by a sudden, excessive electrical discharge from cerebral neurones. The cause is largely unknown but epileptic seizures are associated with cerebral tumours, cerebrovascular disease and head injury.

There are many types of seizures under the classification of epilepsy, but 2 patterns are commonly encountered in the pre-hospital care environment.

Generalised tonic-clonic seizures (grand mal). Generalised seizures cause muscle contraction of the entire body, because both cerebral hemispheres are involved. Loss of consciousness is often the initial phase. The *tonic* phase of the seizure is a violent and rigid fixing of the limbs, with the eyes and head turning to one side. Cyanosis may be evident as respiratory movement is reduced.

The *clonic* phase is a 'jerking' of the body as muscle contraction and spasm occurs. The patient may bite the tongue due to spasm of the tongue and jaw muscles. Breathing may be noisy, with frothy sputum produced. Bladder and bowel control may be lost.

Following the seizure, which usually lasts for about 2 minutes, the patient is unconscious and not responding for a short duration. On regaining consciousness, the patient is often disoriented and confused and may prefer to sleep for several hours.

Absence siezures (petit mal). These are seizures with transient loss of consciousness and characterised by a varying degree of movements, sometimes barely observable. There are four types of absence seizures:

- Absence with increased postural tone. Muscle contraction may give rise to an exaggerated posture, e.g., the head may be thrown back and the patient may walk around with an arched back
- Absence with decreased postural tone. A decrease in muscle tone leads to a slumping of the body and loss of grip. However, it is rare for the patient to fall
- Absence with mild clonus. Twitching of the mouth and rapid blinking, sometimes barely perceptible
- Absence with automatism. Aimless walking, lip licking and swallowing. The seizures are usually of short duration, with the patient momentarily confused, before carrying on quite normally.

Management

Emergency care for epilepsy is aimed at preventing injury during the seizure. Protect the patient from colliding with objects or injuring limbs. The use of a 'bite block' between the teeth to prevent tongue damage is difficult and not advised. In many circumstances, the seizure has passed before the ambulance crew arrives. During the unconscious phase, position the patient to maintain the airway and administer oxygen. Hospitalisation is advisable for further investigation, especially if it is the first seizure experienced by the patient. Transport quietly, offering psychological support.

Status epilepticus is a continuous succession of seizures without any period of recovery. Although not seen frequently outside of institutions, status epilepticus requires urgent medical intervention and is often fatal.

POISONS, DRUGS AND ALCOHOL

A poison is any substance which, when taken into the body in sufficient quantity, either destroys life or seriously impairs body function. Some substances will be harmful in relatively small amounts.

Poisoning may be accidental or deliberate. The major proportion of the accidental poisoning group comprises children in the age group of 6 months to 4 years. Often, poisoning is the result of the careless actions of adults, who leave medications or toxic substances within the reach of children.

Deliberate or intentional poisoning is a frequent form of suicide attempt. Overdose of 'sleeping tablets' and other pharmacological agents is not an uncommon event.

Poisons may enter the body by several means.

Ingestion

The main problems are likely to be:

- Corrosive substances, capable of causing chemical burns, e.g., acids, alkalis, including some household cleaning agents, petroleum products.
- Non corrosive substances, such as tablets and medicines.

Inducing vomiting in corrosive poisoning is *not* indicated.

This may cause further damage if the substance is vomited. Likewise, never induce vomiting in an unconscious patient. Ascertain the history of the poisoning and gather samples to assist in identification. Transport the patient to the emergency department without delay.

Non corrosive substance ingestion may be managed by inducing vomiting. Syrup of Ipecacuanha (Ipecac) is an emetic in general use.

7

However, Ipecac should not be used with adult patients as it is often retained, complicating the poisoning effect. Activated charcoal, which is capable of absorbing 10 times its volume of material is used in some services. Transport the patient expeditiously to the emergency department and if unconscious, maintain airway and respiratory support. Some pharmacological agents may cause respiratory arrest, necessitating ventilation.

Inhalation (gassing)

The effect of inhalational poisoning generally is that of creating an irrespirable atmosphere. The main problems are likely to be:

- Carbon monoxide, a component of motor vehicle exhaust emission and domestic coal gas (not Natural Gas). It combines readily with haemoglobin, thereby reducing the oxygen carrying capacity of the blood
- Common industrial gases including hydrogen sulphide, chlorine, carbon tetrachloride and trichloroethylene, which depress CNS function. Cyanide fumes can rapidly be fatal.

In the management of gas affected patients, it is important to protect yourself.

> **DON'T BECOME A VICTIM BY CARELESS ENTRY**

Establish the nature of the gas and, if safe to do so, remove the patient from the gas-filled environment and administer high flow oxygen.

> **IF A GASSED PATIENT IS NOT BREATHING, VENTILATE BUT DO NOT USE EXPIRED AIR RESUSCITATION**

Transport to the emergency department without delay.

Percutaneous (by absorption directly through the skin)

The main problems are likely to be:

- Insecticides or other substances used in agriculture
- Organophosphate compounds (e.g., malathion and parathion) used in market gardens, orchards and sometimes applied by aerial spraying.

Organophosphates are related to the nerve gases developed for chemical warfare and may enter by ingestion, inhalation or absorption via the skin and/or conjunctiva. They produce, initially, headache, nausea, increased salivation, blurred vision and 'tightness' in the chest.

These effects are usually followed rapidly by vomiting, diarrhoea, severe dyspnoea, loss of consciousness and death, unless treated urgently.

> **DO NOT USE EXPIRED AIR RESUSCITATION FOR ORGANOPHOSPHATE POISONING**

Establish the nature of the compound before commencing treatment. This is vital because some substances will react with oxygen and rapidly become fatal poisonings. Pesticides such as *paraquat* and *diquat* are examples of this group.

Under *no* circumstances should oxygen be administered for paraquat and diquat poisoning.

Immediate contact with poisons information services should be sought and the patient transported to the emergency department rapidly. If oxygen is not contraindicated, ventilate with 100% oxygen and transport without delay.

Percutaneous (by injection or bites)

The main problems are likely to be:

- Injected drugs such as narcotics (heroin or morphine)
- Venom injection from reptiles, spiders or insects.

An overdose of narcotics will cause marked respiratory depression or arrest, hypotension and loss of consciousness. Look for injection sites (track marks) and collect all containers, ampoules and syringes found at the scene.

7

> **TAKE CARE TO AVOID NEEDLE STICK ACCIDENTS**
> **Narcotic abusers may have or carry hepatitis-B and HIV (AIDS)**

Gloves should always be worn for personal protection. Treat the patient with high flow oxygen, with attention to airway maintenance. If respiratory arrest occurs, ventilate with 100% oxygen. IV Narcan will reverse narcotic overdose and should be administered at the scene if it is within your service's protocols. The role of the ambulance officer is patient care and therefore any judgements concerning legal implications are best left to the admitting medical officer in the emergency department.

Venom injection

The factors involved in poisoning by animal venom obviously vary from region to region of the world. The ambulance officer needs to be familiar with local conditions and problems. Australia has one of the largest populations in the world of venomous snakes, which are found throughout the continent.

The majority of snakebites occur on the limbs, particularly the legs. The venom is injected usually deep into the tissues and very little venom is likely to be removed by incising the bite.

The combination of firm pressure over the bite and immobilisation of the limb has been demonstrated to be effective in restricting the venom from entering the bloodstream. A broad bandage, such as a crepe or conforming bandage, applied firmly over the bitten area and covering as much of the limb as possible, plus splinting to steady the limb is the management of choice.

- Do not apply an arterial tourniquet as such methods are no longer recommended
- Do not wash the bitten area, because venom on the skin may help in identifying the snake
- Do not move the patient unnecessarily; if possible, bring the transport to the patient
- Bring the snake to the emergency department only if it can be killed safely
- If the patient exhibits any signs of respiratory distress, administer oxygen and be prepared to ventilate
- Maintain vital signs observations and transport without delay.

The pressure/immobilisation method should not be used for ant, bee and wasp stings unless the patient is known to be highly sensitive to the toxin, as it will prolong the pain. Iced water applied over the site will relieve the sting.

If the patient is allergic to the toxin, apply the pressure/immobilisation technique to reduce the spread of the toxin until examined in the emergency department. Severe reactions may cause respiratory distress and even cardiac arrest. Be prepared to resuscitate the patient and transport without delay.

Insect stings on the head, neck and in the mouth (a frequent occurrence from insects in drink cans and containers), especially in allergic patients, may cause rapid airway impairment. Transport the patient in a sitting position, which will afford airway patency and administer oxygen. Removal to the emergency department should be without delay, but do not panic the patient.

The most common spider found throughout Australia is the redback, clearly identified by the red stripe along the spider's abdomen. There is little treatment necessary in the pre-hospital environment. The application of iced water will provide relief from the pain. As the venom is slow moving, any attempt to restrict it will only increase the pain. However, the venom is potentially lethal and the patient should be transported expeditiously.

The funnel web spider is found mainly on the eastern coast of Australia, predominantly in New South Wales. The venom is rapidly absorbed into the body and has been responsible for many deaths over the years. Treatment should be the same as for snake bite to restrict the venom flow and transport rapidly. An anti-venom is now available for treating the patient.

KNOWLEDGE CHECK

CVA

14. What are the 3 causes of a CVA?

15. Describe what is meant by the term 'transient ischaemic attack'.

16. Describe how you recognise a CVA.

17. What are the important elements of the management of a patient presenting with a CVA?

Diabetic emergencies

18. What are the 2 principal disorders of diabetes?

19. Describe the clinical pictures of the disorders under the headings of history, onset and clinical features.

Epilepsy

20. What are the 2 patterns of seizure commonly encountered in the pre-hospital care environment?

21. What are the important elements of the management of a seizure?

Poisons

22. What are the 4 methods of entry of poisons into the body?

23. Describe the management for each method of poison.

Turn to page 303 to check your answers.

7

FURTHER READING

Buchanan N 1988 Epilepsy and you. Williams & Wilkins, Sydney

Gronwall D, Wrightson P, Waddell P 1990 Head injury the facts: a guide for families and care givers. Oxford University Press, Oxford

Hewson L 1990 When half is whole: my recovery from stroke. Collins Dove, Melbourne

Jennett B, Teasdale G 1981 Management of head injuries. Davis, Philadelphia

Larkins R G 1985 A practical approach to endocrine disorders. Williams & Wilkins, Sydney

Vale J A, Meredith T J 1985 A concise guide to the management of poisoning. Churchill Livingstone, Edinburgh

CHAPTER 8
Approach to trauma

Trauma has been discussed in general in the preceding clinical chapters. The area of musculoskeletal injuries is the focus of this chapter. Special considerations for mass casualty incidents, accessing patients in confined spaces and dealing with entrapment completes the trauma discussion.

Topics covered

Bones and muscles at a glance
The problem of fractured limbs
Mass casualties and the hostile environment
Rescue
Hazardous materials

Any incident, whether acute illness or trauma, requires a systematic approach to ensure that all problems are identified and the correct priority of management is established. The primary, vital signs and secondary surveys discussed in Chapter 2 provide a systematic approach:

- Primary survey—dealing with life threat
- Vital signs survey—to determine the time critical patient
- Secondary survey—the nose-to-toes surface check for injury.

In each of the clinical chapters, specific trauma was described in relation to the effect on major functions. However, a frequently encountered trauma is damage to the body's anatomical framework—the skeleton. Limb injury, in particular, is commonly seen in road crashes and as a result of sporting activities. The relationships between bones and muscles mean that damage to the limbs will usually consist of both fracture and soft tissue injury, with associated bleeding.

8

BONES AND MUSCLES AT A GLANCE

Aim

To develop an understanding of the body framework and skills in managing bone injury

Learning plan

1. **Read the text information**
2. **Supplement reading in anatomy and physiology with a more comprehensive text**
3. **Check your understanding using the knowledge checks**
4. **Practise the skills using the skills guides as a reference to check your competence**

The framework of the body comprises over 200 individual bones, held together by ligaments to form the structure called the skeleton (Fig. 8.1). This structure provides the basic shape and support for the body, affording protection for vital organs (e.g., the skull protects the brain, the rib cage protects the heart and lungs) and enables a wide range of movement.

BONE

Bone is hard connective tissue, composed of organic material (30%), inorganic salts (45%) and water (25%). There are 2 types of bone, compact and cancellous.

Compact bone appears to be solid, but under a microscope can be seen patterns called haversian systems. The most significant structure of these systems is the haversian canal, which runs longitudinally and contains minute blood and lymph vessels, supplying the bone with nutrients.

Cancellous bone has the appearance of a sponge and contains red bone marrow—the blood forming tissue.

Any break in the continuity of the bone (fracture) will result in bleeding. The outer surface of bone is covered by a membrane (periosteum), which provides a protective covering and affords attachment for the muscle tendons.

The bones of the skeleton are classified according to their shape (Figs. 8.2 and 8.3). Long bones, which are greater in length than width, are found in the limbs (e.g., the femur and humerus). Bones of almost equal length and width are classified as short bones (e.g., the bones of the wrist and ankle). Flat bones are relatively thin plates, but provide good protection and vast areas for muscle attachment (e.g., the bones of the skull vault, ribs, scapula and sternum). The fourth classification is irregular bone. These are the bones of complex shape found in the facial area of the skull and the vertebrae of the spine.

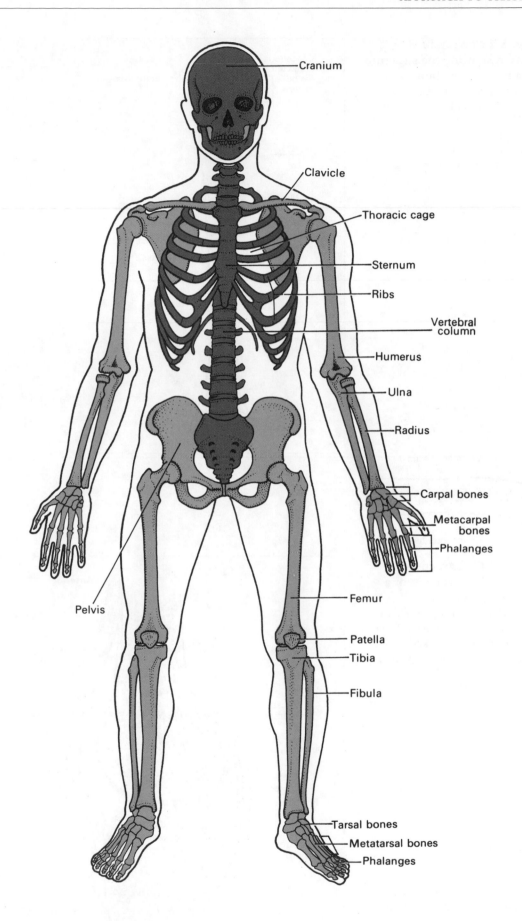

Fig. 8.1 The skeleton. Front view.
(Reproduced with permission from Wilson K J W 1990 Ross & Wilson: Anatomy and physiology in health and illness, 7th edition. Churchill Livingstone, Edinburgh)

Fig. 8.2 Longitudinal section showing the structure of a typical long bone. (Reproduced with permission from Wilson K J W 1990 Ross & Wilson: Anatomy and physiology in health and illness, 7th edition. Churchill Livingstone, Edinburgh)

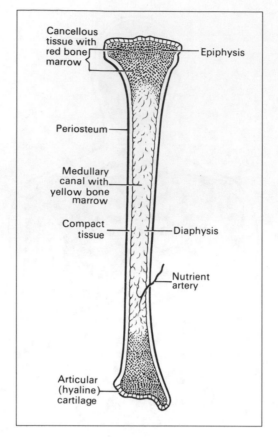

Fig. 8.3 Cross section showing the structure of a typical flat bone. (Reproduced with permission from Wilson K J W 1990 Ross & Wilson: Anatomy and physiology in health and illness, 7th edition. Churchill Livingstone, Edinburgh)

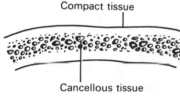

Fig. 8.4 Longitudinal section showing the structure of the knee joint. (Reproduced with permission from Wilson K J W 1990 Ross & Wilson: Anatomy and physiology in health and illness, 7th edition. Churchill Livingstone, Edinburgh)

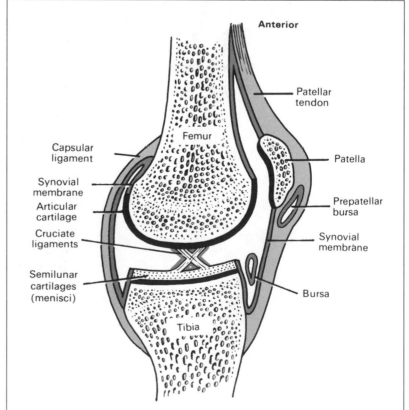

JOINTS

The flexibility and movement of the skeleton is achieved by a variety of joints (articulations), which link the bones to each other. The structure of the joint determines the extent of movement afforded. There are 3 general classifications of joints, synovial, fibrous and cartilaginous.

Synovial joints are articulations in which a space exists between the bones of the joint (Fig. 8.4). They permit varying degrees of movement and are found in all moving areas of the body. The joint is held together by ligaments, which are bands of flexible, slightly elastic fibrous tissue (e.g., the knee).

Fibrous joints are articulations which lack a space between the bones and are held together firmly by fibrous connective tissue (Fig. 8.5), affording little or no movement (e.g., the sutures of the skull).

Fig. 8.5 Cross section showing the structure of a fibrous or fixed joint. (Reproduced with permission from Wilson K J W 1990 Ross & Wilson: Anatomy and physiology in health and illness, 7th edition. Churchill Livingstone, Edinburgh)

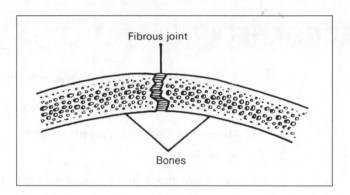

Cartilaginous joints are like the fibrous joint, they are articulations with no space between the bones. Bound together tightly by cartilage, there is again little or no movement afforded (e.g., symphysis pubis).

MUSCLES

The movements of the skeleton are created by the contraction and relaxation of the muscles. Muscle tissue, which accounts for almost 50% of the total body weight, performs 3 functions through its contraction:

- body motion, either total movement (as in running) or localised, such as nodding the head
- posture maintenance, holding the body in a steady position such as sitting or standing
- production of heat, for the maintenance of normal body temperature.

Muscle tissue has 4 key characteristics:

- the ability to receive and respond to stimuli (excitability)
- the ability to shorten and thicken in response to stimuli (contractility)
- the ability to be stretched (extensibility)
- the ability to return to its normal shape following extension or contraction (elasticity).

There are 3 types of muscle tissue: skeletal, smooth and cardiac.

Skeletal muscle is attached to the bones and moves the skeleton. It is known as voluntary muscle because it is under conscious control.

Smooth muscle is found in the walls of hollow structures (e.g., blood vessels and intestines) and known as involuntary muscle—i.e., not under conscious control.

Cardiac muscle is the highly specialised, involuntary muscle mass of the heart.

KNOWLEDGE CHECK

1. What are the 2 types of bone and their structure?

2. What are the 4 classifications of bone?

3. Name the 3 general classifications of joints and give an example of each.

4. What are the 3 functions of muscle tissue?

5. Describe the 3 types of muscle tissue.

Turn to page 304 to check your answers.

THE PROBLEM OF FRACTURED LIMBS

Determining the presence of bone injury depends on gathering a history of the incident including the injury mechanisms and an examination of the body surface.

The type of incident in which the patient was involved, will provide valuable information to help identify probable bone injury. If the patient was struck by a solid object or fell from a height, the forces created by the impact may have been sufficient to fracture bones. In some cases, the patient may report feeling something 'snapping'.

Direct violence may result in bone fracture at the point of contact (e.g., a pedestrian struck by the bumper of a car or a limb struck by a heavy object). Indirect violence may cause a fracture some distance from the point of contact, such as a hip fracture following the knee colliding forcefully with the dashboard in a motor vehicle, or a base of skull fracture from landing heavily on the feet in a fall). Elderly people whose bones are brittle may suffer fractures, especially of the neck of femur, from quite minimal force. These are referred to as *pathologic* fractures and may also occur as a result of diseases in the bone. Muscle contraction of a violent nature occurring in seizures may also produce bone injury.

A significant feature of fractures is well localised pain (at the site of injury). The physical examination, particularly of the extremities, is made easier by comparing the opposite limb, which normally has the same shape. Check the injured limb against the other for evidence of deformity, unnatural position and shortening. Gently feel the site for irregularity of the bone. If the limb is moved, which is only during the splinting procedure, a grating sound or crepitus may be heard as the broken bone fragments grind against each other. However, this must not be deliberately sought, because it may cause further injury.

The patient may complain of tenderness around the site, which is usually discoloured (early bruising) and swollen. Inability to move the limb is another feature. Check the limb for loss of sensation (suggesting nervous impairment due to the fracture) and palpate a distal pulse. The absence of circulation or sensation will require the use of gentle traction along the limb to reduce the compression of blood vessels and nerves.

8

Summary of clinical features—fractures

- Pain at the site of injury
- Irregularity, deformity and shortening
- Loss of movement or use of the limb
- Swelling of tissues at the site
- Discolouration of surrounding tissues
- Unnatural position
- Crepitus or a grating of bone fragments
- Tenderness at the site of injury.

Dislocations occur when the injury involves a joint. The features are often identical to those of a fracture and for this reason are treated as a fracture.

There are several classifications of fracture, but these are of little significance in pre-hospital care because closed fractures cannot be seen. More importantly, the presence of a wound at the site of the fracture (open fracture) or the protrusion of bone ends through the skin, will require dressing before splinting the limb. If the bone protrudes, *do not* attempt to force it back by traction as this will contaminate the site and may cause further injury.

If the limb is angulated (twisted in a bizarre manner), it can be straightened, providing the site *does not involve a joint and is on a single bone* (shaft of femur or humerus). Before using the straightening technique, analgesia should be administered.

Straightening an angulated limb

- Support the proximal end of the limb above the site
- Grip the distal end of the limb (at the wrist or ankle) and apply downward traction
- If resistance is felt or the patient reports too much discomfort, stop immediately and immobilise the limb in the position found

The management of fractures is a lower priority in the total care of the patient. Because the patient is reporting severe pain at the fracture site, there is a tendency to be attracted to this injury before considering the more important aspects of total care. While the injury may be quite painful, it does not pose a threat to life and should not be attended to until the higher priorities are managed.

SPLINTING

Immobilisation of fractured limbs can be achieved by 2 methods:

- anatomical splinting—securing the limb to a part of the body (e.g., tying the legs together or securing the arm to the body).
- mechanical splinting—applying a specially designed rigid device to the injured limb.

The aim of splinting is to prevent movement of the limb to reduce further injury and pain.

Principles of splinting

- Administer analgesia before splinting
- Splint before moving the patient
  (this may be modified if the patient's life is in danger)
- Assess distal circulation and sensation before *and* after splinting.
- Immobilise the joint *above and below* the fracture site
- Control bleeding and dress open fractures before splinting
- If in doubt, always treat as a fracture.

Traction splints

Traction splinting was first developed on the battlefields of World War I. The Thomas traction splint was a solid metal frame on to which a traction system was applied by means of a bottle knot around the ankle and a windlass tie or weights to achieve traction.

Today modern traction splints achieve traction through mechanical means. There are 2 splints commonly used in emergency care. The Hare splint (Fig. 8.6) and a relatively new design called the Donway splint (Fig. 8.7). Despite the improvements of modern technology, the basic principle of the Thomas splint survives.

8

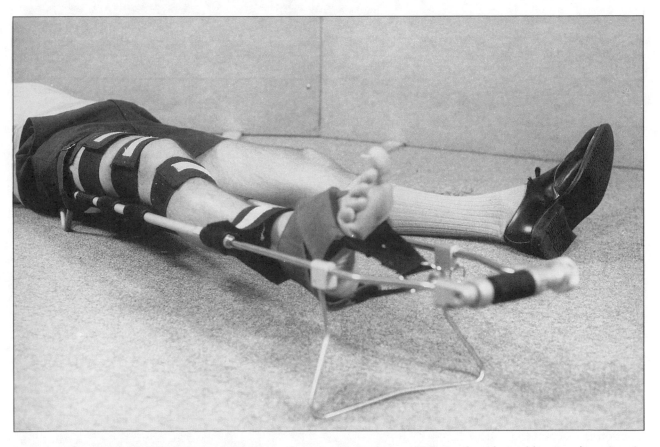

Fig. 8.6 The Hare traction splint applied for a fracture of the femur. Ensure that the ankle strap is correctly applied to maintain effective traction.

The main use of traction splinting is to immobilise fractures of the shaft of femur, where muscle action tends to cause impaction of the broken bone ends or an overriding of the break. In-line reduction of this tension reduces further damage to surrounding tissues and provides rigid support for one of the most significant and serious bone injuries. Traction splints may be used for fractures below the knee (except the ankle and foot) provided traction is not applied.

Fracture of femur, because it is the largest long bone of the skeleton, causes extensive bleeding into the tissues and will result in significant hypovolaemia.

TASKS

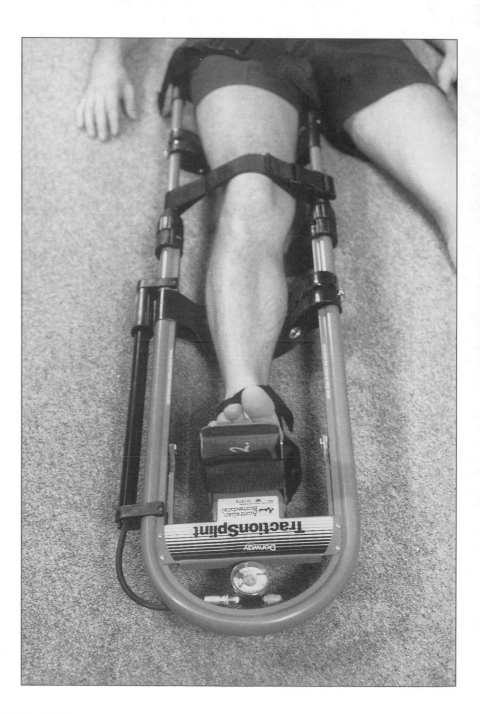

Fig. 8.7 The Donway traction splint operates by pneumatic pressure. Once traction is reached the collets are locked, and the pressure is released.

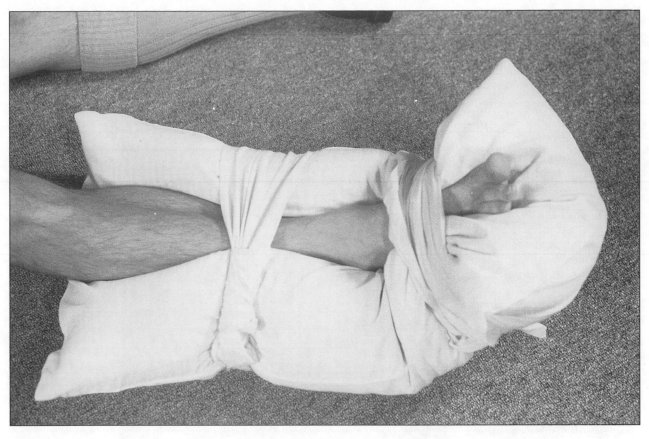

Fig. 8.8 A pillow makes a useful improvised splint since it conforms to the shape of the limb.

Fractures to the ankle or foot can be effectively immobilised using a pillow as a splint (Fig. 8.8). An advantage of this technique is that the pillow conforms to the shape and position of the ankle and foot. If the fracture constricts the blood supply or nerves to the foot, evidenced by loss of sensation or lack of distal pulses and a cold pale extremity, the limb can be easily manipulated and resecured in the pillow.

Air splints (inflatable) have been used extensively in pre-hospital care for many years. However, their major disadvantage is susceptibility to puncture, especially in the road crash setting, where glass fragments are often around the patient. If air splints are used, remember the principle of immobilising the joint above and below the fracture site. Therefore, in most cases, the full arm and full leg splints are the only suitable devices (Fig. 8.9). Air splints are also useful in retaining dressings and as an aid in the control of bleeding.

Upper limb fractures should be left in the position in which they are found. The simplest method is to secure the limb either to, or across, the body. The use of arm slings in pre-hospital care, especially in the ambulance environment, is limited by the fact that most patients require transport by stretcher and no real purpose is served by their application. The use of a pillow to support upper limb fractures, especially those of the forearm is effective and affords excellent comfort for the patient.

8

TASKS	1. Pillow splint applied to an ankle and foot	288
	2. Air splint applied to a leg and an arm	289–290

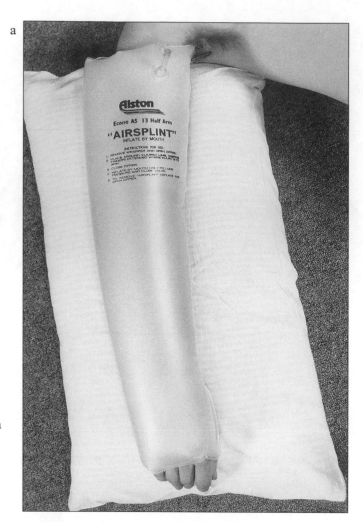

Fig. 8.9 Air splints applied to *a* the arm and *b* the leg. In an environment where these splints can be kept fully inflated, they are useful for immobilising fractures and retaining dressings in place.

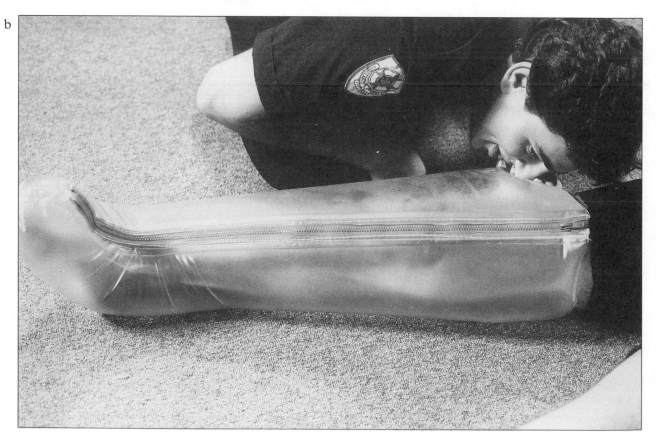

KNOWLEDGE CHECK

6. Describe how the 3 causes of fractures occur.

7. What are the 10 clinical features of fractures?

8. What are the steps in straightening an angulated limb?

9. What are the 2 methods of immobilising fractured limbs?

10. What are the 6 principles of splinting?

Turn to page 304 to check your answers.

MASS CASUALTIES AND THE HOSTILE ENVIRONMENT

Aim

To develop an understanding of the response to major incidents and the hostile environment

Learning plan

1. Read the text information
2. Check your service's major incident plan (DISPLAN) for local procedures and orders
3. Check your local environment and make a list of hazardous goods stored in or transported through your area

Emergency responses to trauma, whether they be to road traffic crashes, industrial accidents or in the home or school yard, generally involve one or a few victims. The strategies for dealing with these incidents are the standards upon which the ambulance officer normally functions. However, in events involving many casualties, e.g., multiple car crashes, aircraft and rail crashes, or natural disasters such as earthquakes and cyclones, the strategies must be altered to cope as quickly and effectively as possible.

8

THE FIRST RESPONDERS

The role of the first ambulance crew at the incident is to establish some order. This is vital preparation for the collection, treatment and transport of casualties.

It is not possible to devote time to one casualty who requires extensive resuscitation measures, when several others can be saved with relatively minor care. If the incident is to be managed effectively, there is a need to establish, as early as possible, the resources that will be required.

One member of the crew must take the first responsibility for sorting and organising the casualties. This crew member is known as the *Casualty collecting officer* (CCO). The sorting task firstly involves identifying the number of stretcher casualties (those who will require transport by stretcher) and the number of walking wounded. This must be communicated by radio so that the necessary additional resources can be marshalled.

Treatment is limited to life support first aid (ABCs)—clear airways and position casualties. If there are bystanders at the scene, they can be of great assistance by helping with simple first aid measures and carrying the casualties until trained personnel arrive.

A suitable site for collecting the casualties should be found. Gathering the casualties to a single point, if possible, makes the task of sorting and treating easier to manage. Sorting now involves the process of 'triage'. This is the classification of casualties into 4 groups:

- Those requiring urgent treatment—top priority
- Those who are stable and can be delayed for a short time— second priority
- Those requiring first aid treatment only
- The dead.

If the casualties are spread widely and it is not possible to gather them to a single site, divide the scene into areas with other collecting sites.

When ambulance crews and medical teams arrive, direct them to the most urgent casualties. The walking wounded should be kept at the collecting point and not transported to the hospital as they will tend to overwhelm the emergency department.

The second member of the first responding crew must assume the responsibility for controlling the resources upon their arrival—*Transport control officer* (TCO). A loading point, with clear access and egress, should be selected close to the casualty collecting point. If there are large numbers of ambulances responding, a holding point should be selected to reduce the possibility of congestion at the loading area. These locations must be advised by radio.

The access and egress routes must be kept clear of other traffic. Police assistance may be required. Use bystanders to help until the arrival of the police.

The TCO should then ensure that ambulances are loaded efficiently, record casualty details and despatch the ambulances to suitable hospitals—not all to the same hospital as this may overwhelm the emergency department.

Incidents which take considerable time to resolve, involve a large response, or escalate, will require a scene *coordinator*. This is usually a senior officer whose responsibility it is to oversee the ambulance activities at the scene. The coordinator must ensure that the CCO and TCO know that he or she has taken command and that all directions for ambulance tasks at the scene are through the coordinator (Fig. 8.10).

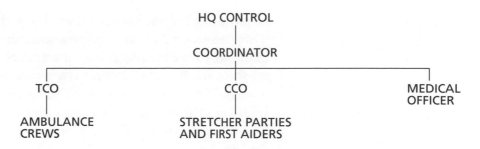

Fig. 8.10 The chain of command for major incidents.

The coordinator is responsible for liaising with other emergency services and combating authorities and should be located at the scene *command point*. If a medical officer is at the scene, all requests for transport of casualties must still be made through the coordinator. The maintenance of communications with the CCO, TCO and headquarters control is essential in managing the scene to greatest efficiency and, along with the first responding crew, the coordinator should be the last to leave the scene.

TERRORIST INCIDENTS

An unfortunate reality of the modern world is the occurence of terrorist attacks. Once these events were mainly against military targets. However, in recent times, terrorist activities have also turned towards 'soft' targets—the general public—by attacks on public buildings and sniper assaults in the streets. An attack is not always the work of an organisation, incited by political or religious conflict. Often, incidents are the acts of individuals. Regardless of the motives behind these events, the ambulance officer is required to respond to the victims of bomb explosions and other shooting incidents. Many responses are often to an active incident.

> **APPROACH ALL TERRORIST INCIDENTS WITH CAUTION AND SEEK ADVICE ABOUT SAFE AREAS BEFORE ENTERING THE DANGER ZONE**

The management of victims of ballistic injuries differs little from managing blunt and penetrating trauma as discussed in earlier chapters. However, the extent of the trauma is frequently widespread, with multiple injuries. Blast effects from explosions may produce serious injury to the internal organs and many victims will be classified as time critical patients. Single ballistic injuries (gunshot wounds) may often appear to be simple wounds. However, consider the effects of a high velocity missile striking the body. The energy of the missile is dispersed through the tissues in shock waves, similar to the concentric ripples on the surface of a pond when you throw a stone into the water. This 'tissue quake' may destroy structures some distance from the entry site of the missile. Look for evidence of damage in body regions adjacent to the entry wound. Be aware of the likelihood of an exit wound. An entry wound in the anterior chest wall is usually quite small, but the exit site in the posterior chest wall may be significant. The degree of destruction depends on the velocity of the missile and the distance of the weapon. The identification of the type of weapon and calibre of the missile, along with an estimation of the range, is useful information to pass on to the emergency department. These data may assist the surgeon in early identification of the extent of injury and the urgency of initial hospital care.

RESCUE

The principal role of the ambulance officer is patient care. In some circumstances, access to the patient and retrieval is difficult, necessitating rescue and extrication. While some ambulance services perform a rescue role, the provision of heavy rescue is the province of the fire department or other combating authority. Therefore the focus of rescue in this text is limited to gaining simple access and becoming aware of the hazards at the scene.

The assessment of the scene is the crucial factor. The rescue of people trapped in motor vehicles is the most common rescue incident encountered by the ambulance officer. While the complete removal of the roof provides easier access to the patient and a large area for emergency care, it also introduces hazards of sharp metal, and an open door may suffice.

Don't ignore the obvious.

Check the doors of the vehicle before you call in the heavy cutting equipment—unnecessary delay may be avoided.

If cutting equipment is required to gain access to the patient or to facilitate extrication, minimising further risks to the patient is vital. Protect the patient as much as possible by shielding them with a blanket. Liaise with the rescue personnel to ensure the methods employed are safe and the most suitable.

Moving the patient from the wreckage often poses problems because of multiple injuries and limited space through which to lift. Many devices have been developed to facilitate lifting and extrication—e.g., the Kendrik Extrication Device (KED). While most of these devices are well designed and provide an effective means of protecting and lifting the patient, there is a more readily available and versatile device, carried in every ambulance—the blanket. It can be folded (or rolled if required) and slipped under or around the patient without causing unnecessary movement. Lifting and moving the patient is then easier and, if care is taken to ensure the blanket is held firmly, in-line body support for most injuries will be maintained.

ELECTRICAL HAZARDS

Electrical hazards are a frequent concern in road traffic crashes. Vehicles colliding with power poles can bring wires down. Overhead power systems are protected by circuit breakers, but because they are affected by climatic conditions, lightning and tree branches, the systems are also fitted with automatic 'reclose devices'. When a fault occurs on a line, the protecting device opens for a few seconds and recloses to maintain power (some are programmed to open and reclose several times). Therefore, in some cases, a wire can be down but still alive. It cannot be said with certainty that a wire lying on the ground is not dangerous, or what its voltage may be. Stray voltage in the ground near a 'downed' live wire can also prove fatal.

> **ASSUME ALL WIRES ARE LIVE AND HIGH VOLTAGE. THE MINIMUM SAFETY CLEARANCE IS AT LEAST 2 METRES**

CONFINED SPACES

Confined spaces are another potentially hazardous situation. Any location where natural ventilation may be restricted (vats, pipes, trenches, or containers which contain or have contained harmful fumes) should be approached with extreme caution. Entering a confined space without adequate protection places the rescuer at risk, because unaided human senses cannot detect lack of oxygen, some noxious fumes or explosive atmospheres until it is too late.

Oxygen deficiency is the most common hazard; e.g., oxygen deficiency tests conducted by the University of Melbourne demonstrate that the rusting of a closed steel tank (in a damp atmosphere) will reduce the available oxygen in the air to a dangerous level in about 5 days. If an oxidising agent is introduced (sea air), the time is reduced to approximately 5 hours. An unlined steel tank at a reservoir or industrial site could become lethal overnight.

> **DO NOT ATTEMPT RESCUES FROM CONFINED SPACES WITHOUT SELF-CONTAINED BREATHING APPARATUS**

8

STEEP DESCENTS

Rescue situations, from time to time, involve steep descents to reach a patient who has fallen over a cliff or steep culvert. The first consideration, which applies always to any incident, is personal safety, especially if you are unsure of, or not skilled in descent techniques.

**IF YOU ARE NOT SKILLED, DO NOT ATTEMPT RESCUE.
SUMMON EXPERT HELP**

Most ambulance stretchers are not designed for use in rescue settings, especially steep descent. One of the most effective stretchers developed for use in difficult situations is the Paraguard stretcher (Fig. 8.11). Developed in the UK by the PQ Parachute Company, it is a light, strong, easily assembled device, providing a wide range of alternatives for extrication. When the Paraguard is applied, the patient is secure, comfortable and well supported. A variety of safe lifting points enables the stretcher to be carried as a normal stretcher and raised or lowered vertically, as well as by a 4-point suspension sling.

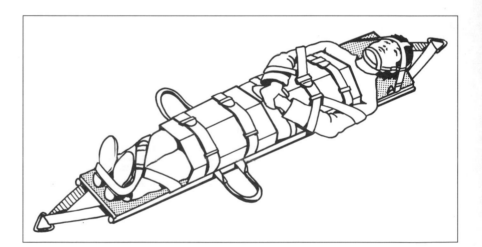

Fig. 8.11 The Paraguard stretcher is specially designed for extrication involving confined spaces or steep descents.

HAZARDOUS MATERIALS

A modern society relies heavily on synthetic materials and petroleum products. Industrial complexes are a part of every major city, producing vast quantities of products used in almost every facet of our lives. The chemicals necessary for production, the products and waste materials are transported daily by road and rail tankers. In recent years, greater awareness of the potential for widespread damage and loss of life from serious accidents has developed. Major spillages, fires in storage and transport depots, and tanker accidents on our roads occur frequently.

Responding to incidents involving hazardous materials increases the risks to all emergency personnel. Contamination can prove, and has proved to be, fatal, necessitating greater understanding of safety procedures and provision of protective clothing.

> **EXTREME CAUTION IS REQUIRED WHEN CHEMICAL HAZARD EXIST OR IS SUSPECTED**

Identification of the substance is essential *before* starting any emergency care.

Government legislation requires that all hazardous goods be clearly identified by signs and information panels. Road and rail vehicles must display information panels on both sides of the vehicle and separate containers are also required to display the nature of the material contained. The information panel (Fig. 8.12) displays:

- The chemical *name*
- The *principal danger* associated with the substance (displayed in a diamond symbol or class label). In some cases a secondary risk label will also be included
- The *UN substance number* (a 4-digit number allocated to a substance, based on a listing given in 'Transport of Dangerous Goods' (United Nations 1970) and its subsequent amendments. This number applies to only one chemical and therefore it is uniquely characterised. The use of the number simplifies the relaying of identification of chemicals with complex names

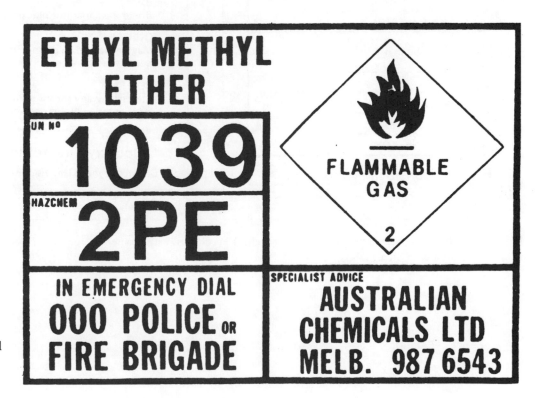

Fig. 8.12 A typical Hazchem information panel.

- The *HAZCHEM code* (a 2 or 3 digit alpha-numeric code) indicating the action required in the event of spillage or accident. This code was developed by the London Fire Brigade
- *Emergency service assistance* contact telephone number for notification of police and fire services
- *Specialist advice* telephone number for assistance to emergency personnel including on-site help with special equipment.

The HAZCHEM code does not require specific knowledge of chemicals or reference to a textbook. The interpretation of the code is made by reference to a scale and notes (Fig. 8.13), which should be either a sticker fixed to the interior of the ambulance, or a card carried by the ambulance officer.

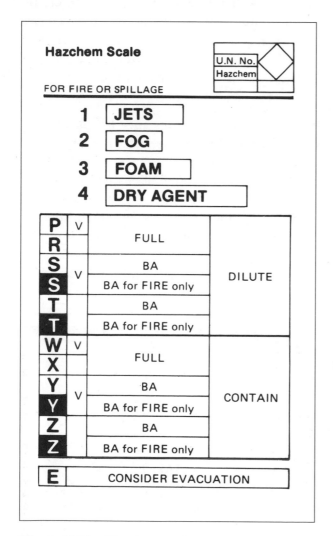

Notes for Guidance

FOG
In the absence of fog equipment a fine spray may be used.

DRY AGENT
Water **must not** be allowed to come into contact with the substance at risk.

V
Can be violently or even explosively reactive.

FULL
Full body protective clothing with BA.

BA
Breathing apparatus plus protective gloves.

DILUTE
May be washed to drain with large quantities of water.

CONTAIN
Prevent, by any means available, spillage from entering drains or water course.

———

Country Fire Authority 1981.

© Crown copyright UK. Reprinted by permission

Fig. 8.13 The Hazchem scale. (Crown copyright. Reproduced with the permission of the Controller of Her Majesty's Stationery Office (UK))

The scale consists of 3 sections.

The numbers at the top indicate which fire-fighting medium is to be used. The letters in the middle (black on white, and white on black) key into the three columns on the right, which are explained in the notes. If present, 'E' as shown at the bottom of the scale means evacuation should be considered as a first priority. The extent and necessity for evacuation will depend on the location and amount of the spillage.

Using the example shown in Figure 8.12, the HAZCHEM code 2PE is interpreted:

2 = water, fog, or spray for fire fighting.
P = (V) violent reaction is possible, full protection with BA is required and the hazard may be diluted.
E = consider evacuation.

The ambulance officer, on arrival at an incident involving hazardous materials, must firstly establish a safe working zone. This should be no closer than 70 metres from the hazard. If other combating agencies are present at the scene (fire service or police), a safety perimeter will already be established. Do not enter the area until the combating agency declares the hazard contained and the area safe to proceed.

Patients involved in a chemical spillage may be contaminated and before commencing emergency care, their decontamination is essential. This procedure is normally carried out by the fire service. If the combating authority requires the ambulance crew to enter the hazard zone to manage the patients, full protective clothing must be used. However, it is better to remain outside of the zone and set up a treatment area adjacent to the decontamination point. It is extremely difficult to manage patient care procedures when dressed in a full protective suit.

FURTHER READING

8

Crawford-Adams J, Hamblen D 1990 Outline of orthopaedics. Churchill Livingstone, Edinburgh

Huckstep R L 1982 A simple guide to trauma. Churchill Livingstone, Edinburgh

Moore R E 1991 Vehicle rescue and extrication. Mosby, St. Louis

CHAPTER 9
Advanced life support

The concept of advanced life support (ALS) is not new. In fact, if one considers its definition, 'the use of invasive techniques and pharmacological agents', then ALS has been practised by ambulance officers since the introduction of analgesics in the early 1960s. However the term ALS has become widely used to refer to those procedures and protocols beyond the general definition of basic life support.

In Australia ALS developments occurred in the late 1960s and early 1970s. Mobile coronary care, mobile intensive care or 'paramedic' ambulances, crewed by specially trained officers, are today operating in most States.

In preceding chapters, several procedures which by definition are within the realm of ALS were covered. Those procedures could be argued as being an integral part of today's modern pre-hospital standards, rather than essentially extended care.

The purpose of this chapter is to provide a further exploration of a range of procedures which can be applied to pre-hospital patient management.

Topics covered

Airway support
Chest auscultation
Chest decompression
Drug administration
Common pharmacological agents.

9

Aim

To develop an understanding of a range of extended skills in the management of respiratory problems

Learning plan

1. **Read the text information**
2. **Practise using the skills guides to check your competence**

AIRWAY SUPPORT

In some situations of airway obstruction, manual methods such as gravity, finger probes and back blows, may not dislodge the foreign body from the upper airway. An additional method is the use of a laryngoscope as a lighted spatula to inspect the upper airway and Magill forceps to grip and remove the object once seen.

In the emergency environment, there is little need for a sophisticated laryngoscope with detachable blades. A single-piece unit, with a fixed blade incorporated in the handle is probably more practical. The most important feature of any laryngoscope is the capacity for good illumination at the tip of the blade.

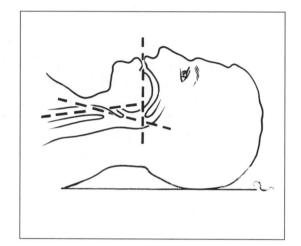

Fig. 9.1 The normal alignment of the airway showing the 3 planes: oropharynx, laryngopharynx and trachea.

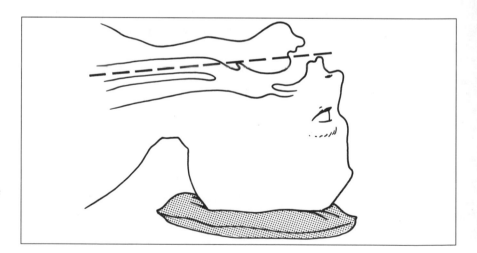

Fig. 9.2 The sniffing position which eliminates the angles of the airway, facilitating direct vision to the vocal chords.

MANAGING AN IMPACTED FOREIGN BODY

The correct positioning of the patient's head is a crucial step in visualising the upper airway. The normal anatomical alignment consists of three planes (Fig. 9.1). The sniffing position eliminates the angles and facilitates a direct line of vision to the vocal cords. It consists of two key points—*flexion* of the neck and *extension* of the head. A folded towel, about 5 cm thick, placed under the patient's head will create the desired flexion (Fig. 9.2).

All laryngoscopes are designed for left hand use. Hold the laryngoscope with the handle in the palm of the left hand, the fingers supporting the handle with a light grip. Do not wrap the thumb around the handle, as this will alter the direction of force when power is applied to lift the tongue. The power grip is applied by exerting gentle pressure with a push in the direction of the handle, with the thumb parallel to the handle (Fig. 9.3). This technique will eliminate angulation of the blade, which may result in damage to the teeth and/or mucosa. Using a single size fixed blade for both adult and paediatric patients requires care. Insert only the first third of the blade when inspecting the airway of a paediatric patient.

Magill forceps are designed for use with the laryngoscope. The offset handle affords direct vision along the laryngoscope blade during use. The expanded ends of the forceps eliminate the risk of traumatising tissues in the airway during insertion and the grooved inner surfaces ensure a firm grip of the object.

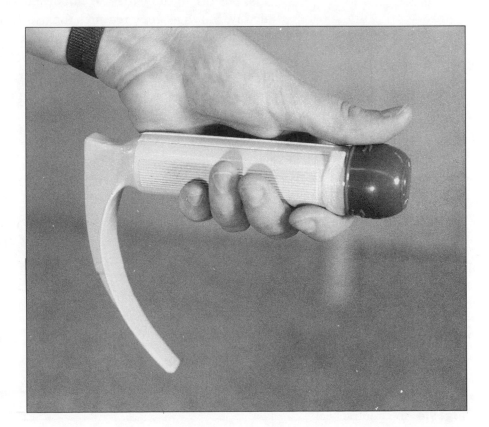

Fig. 9.3 The correct grip of the laryngoscope. The thumb in line with the handle helps keep the blade straight.

9

ENDOTRACHEAL INTUBATION

In most circumstances, the patient's airway can be effectively managed by posture, suction and the insertion of an oropharyngeal airway. However, when these measures fail, or if there is a need to secure the airway so that other procedures may be more effectively managed, the method of choice is endotracheal intubation or ETI (Fig. 9.4). The advantages of this technique are:

- The airway is protected from aspiration of gastric contents by a cuffed tube in the trachea
- The technique maintains a clear air pathway
- IPPV with 100% oxygen can be achieved without the risk of gastric distension
- It facilitates tracheal suctioning.

If the procedure is performed correctly, misplacement of the tube will be avoided (i.e. into the oesophagus or inserted too deeply, which results in intubation of the right bronchus).

Prior to intubating, it is vital to ventilate the patient adequately, via a bag-mask system, with supplemental oxygen. This will begin the essential management of hypoxia and provide some oxygen support necessary during the 20 seconds of the intubation procedure. Ventilation can be performed while the equipment for tubing is being prepared.

There are several essential tasks required before attempting ETI. The posture of the patient is important to achieve a clear view of the airway. Laryngoscopy requires the use of the sniffing position, which effectively reduces the normal anatomical alignment of the airway.

All equipment for the intubation procedure and subsequent ventilation of the patient must be prepared to minimise the time delay in resuming ventilation. The most appropriate size endotracheal tube

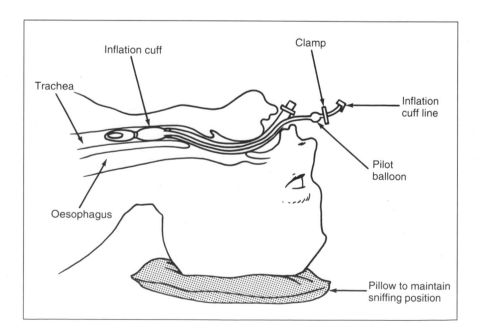

Fig. 9.4 An endotracheal tube in position.

must be selected. Normally, an 8 mm or 8.5 mm (internal diameter) tube will be appropriate for most adult patients. Tube sizes for paediatric patients vary from 2.5 mm to 7.5 mm (internal diameter) depending on the age of the child. The smaller tubes are uncuffed. Before the tube is inserted, the cuffed end should be lubricated to prevent mucosal damage during entry into the airway.

Placement of the tube must always be under *direct vision* with the vocal cords in view. If the cords cannot be visualised, tubing should not be attempted, because invariably this 'blind' approach results in the oesophagus being intubated and precious time is lost.

Once the patient is intubated, which should take no more than 20 seconds, the chest should be checked for evidence of equal lung inflation. This is done by ventilating the patient and observing chest movements. Auscultation of the chest (by stethoscope) should be performed to ensure that breath sounds are equal and audible on both sides. If no breath sounds are audible, the tube is not in the trachea and should be removed and re-inserted after adequate ventilation of the patient. If breath sounds are absent on one side of the chest, the tube is in the right bronchus. This can be easily remedied by gently pulling the tube upwards while ventilating the patient and listening for return of sounds in the quiet lung field. Once audible, secure the tube in position.

CHEST AUSCULTATION

Auscultation means listening for sounds. The most important body sounds to consider in advanced pre-hospital emergency care are those of respiration.

Auscultation is aided by the use of a stethoscope, which normally has 2 amplifying components to detect sounds of different frequency. The flat diaphragm component will detect high frequency sounds when held firmly against the skin. This is suited to detection of lung sounds and checking equality of air entry following endotracheal intubation. The reverse amplifying component is a bell shape, used to detect low frequency sounds (e.g., heart and abdominal sounds).

Normal lung sounds consist of 2 types, breath and vocal.

Breath sounds are produced in the airways and the intensity of the sound is related to the total airflow at the mouth and in the lung regions. Therefore, a reduction in intensity suggests obstruction to airflow.

Vocal sounds are laryngeal sounds transmitted through the airways to the chest wall.

Abnormal lung sounds, previously classified by terms such as rhonci, rales and crepitations, are more simply divided into wheezes and crackles.

9

Wheezes are a musical whistling sound produced by the continuous vibration of the opposing walls of the airway. The frequency of wheezes is dependent upon the airflow and the physical properties of the airway walls. This sound suggests significant narrowing of the small airways.

Crackles may sound course or fine. Alveolar dysfunction produces a late inspiratory crackle, and early crackles heard during either the inspiratory or expiratory phases suggests small airways disease.

CHEST DECOMPRESSION

Injury to the thorax may result in lung injury and air escaping into the pleural cavity (pneumothorax). If the laceration of the lung wall creates a 'flutter valve' effect, (i.e., on inspiration air enters the pleural space, and on exhalation, the air is trapped by closure of the laceration), a tension pneumothorax may develop. The increased tension in the pleural cavity causes lung collapse and compression of the sound lung, further reducing respiratory function. If the tension is not relieved quickly, respiratory failure may occur and the chances of survival for the patient are markedly reduced.

NEEDLE THORACOTOMY

A life-saving procedure, needle thoracotomy requires *confirmation* of the presence of a tension pneumothorax as a *prerequisite*. This is achieved by inserting a 23G needle, attached to a syringe containing sterile water or normal saline. The site for insertion is the 2nd intercostal space, in the mid-clavicular line, on the affected side of the thorax (Fig. 9.5). To prevent infection, the site must be swabbed before inserting the needle.

The needle is inserted at 90° to the chest, immediately above the margin of the 3rd rib, to avoid thoracic nerves and blood vessels. Once the needle is fully inserted, the syringe plunger is withdrawn and the fluid observed for evidence of air bubbling. If air bubbles through the fluid, a tension pneumothorax is confirmed and the needle can be withdrawn and replaced by a wide bore needle (e.g., 14G Bardi-cath or an equivalent) to commence decompression of the chest.

A flutter valve, to prevent re-entry of air through the needle, can be created by cutting the end of the Bardi-cath plastic sleeve (Fig. 9.6). An alternative is to attach a portion of a surgical glove finger to the hub of the needle.

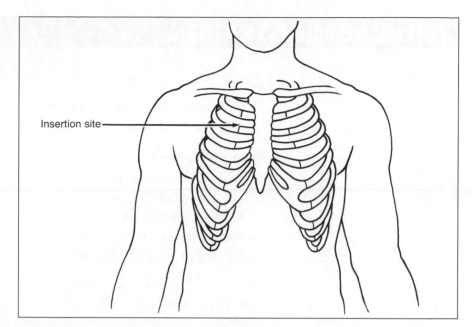

Fig. 9.5 The insertion site for needle thoracotomy in the 2nd intercostal space immediately above the 3rd rib to avoid nerves and blood vessels.

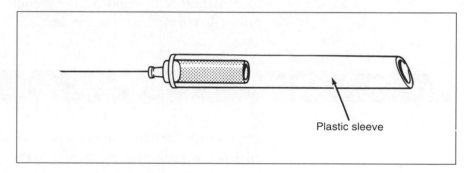

Fig. 9.6 A flutter valve can be made using the Bardi-cath and cutting the plastic sleeve.

The needle is inserted in the same site as used in the confirming procedure, after swabbing the site again. The needle must be taped securely in place and the patient re-assessed for improved respiratory status. Transport to the emergency department should be then undertaken without further delay.

During transport, check for air movement after 5 minutes. If there is no air movement through the needle and valve, remove the needle and dress the site. If the patient's respiratory status deteriorates and there is evidence again of tension, the procedure should be repeated.

Invasive procedures such as needle thoracotomy should never be attempted in a moving vehicle.

Stop the ambulance to ensure that there is no risk of accidental needle stick to both the patient and the ambulance officer.

TASK	Needle thoracotomy	296

DRUG ADMINISTRATION

Aim

To develop an understanding of common pharmacological agents used in pre-hospital care

Learning plan

1. Read the text information
2. Check your service's policies and the medico-legal requirements for drug administration
3. Check your service's protocols for the appropriate dosage and procedure for administration of the drugs

The use of intravenous drugs in pre-hospital care is largely related to managing chest pain and the associated cardiac arrythmias. The protocols for their use vary according to the ambulance service's medical authorities and advisory bodies and therefore no specific protocols are presented in this text.

PHARMACOLOGY

Drug administration for the treatment of disease dates back to the ancient civilizations of Egypt and Arabia. Many of the remedies were known to people who had no medical training and were used in the household, often in a misdirected fashion. It was not until an understanding of physiology and pathology emerged in the 19th century that the uses and effects of drugs were studied scientifically. The discovery of chemical structures and alteration to chemical composition enabled the development of drugs whose actions were known through chemical analysis and refined to limit side effects. Despite the voluminous research, the way in which many drug effects are produced remains largely unknown. However 3 generally known effects are antimetabolic, enzyme inhibition and receptor interference.

Antimetabolites are similar to nutritional substances used by cells. The cell cannot distinguish between the genuine nutritional substance and the antimetabolite, whose action is to stop the cell multiplying. An example of this type of drug is an antibiotic, which stops the growth of bacteria.

Enzyme inhibitors prevent the actions of the body's enzymes responsible for the various chemical processes. For example, diuretic drugs inhibit the enzymes required for the reabsorption of water and salts, causing them to pass through the kidneys and be excreted.

Receptor interference. The surface of some body cells contain indentations and other structures known as receptors. Certain substances, which are produced in the body (e.g., hormones), link into the receptor and stimulate a cell response; e.g., acetylcholine stimulates muscle fibres to contract. Certain drugs will link into the receptors and produce either a stimulus similar to the naturally produced substance or block the action; e.g., atropine will block acetylcholine stimulation.

INTRAVENOUS DRUG ADMINISTRATION

A safe and efficient practice for drug administration is the establishment of an intravenous fluid pathway. The IV line affords a direct access for immediate use and should further drugs be required later in the emergency department, when poor perfusion may make peripheral vein cannulation difficult.

The commonly used fluid to keep an IV line open is 5% dextrose, an isotonic crystalloid solution. Dextrose, composed of sugar (5% dextrose) and water, is a safe solution with all patients, but excessive administration will cause a fluid overload and may result in pulmonary oedema.

Volume-depleted patients require fluid replacement which contains electrolytes to restore the body's chemical balance. The use of volume expanding fluids in pre-hospital care is limited to solutions which can be carried in the ambulance and are not affected by moderate extremes of temperature. Haemaccel (polygeline) is in general use in pre-hospital care and is an isotonic colloid solution. It increases the volume of the intravascular compartment and raises the plasma colloid osmotic pressure, thus improving tissue perfusion.

Compound sodium lactate (Hartmann's solution), is an isotonic crystalloid solution, also used for volume-depleted patients and is composed of electrolytes in a similar concentration to extracellular fluid. If no other fluid is available, it may be used to keep a vein open and for the administration of drugs, but should be replaced as soon as possible by 5% dextrose.

COMMON PHARMACOLOGICAL AGENTS

9

A variety of drugs are used in pre-hospital emergency care. Doses may vary according to local medical authorities and for this reason, dosage ranges in this text are presented as a general guide.

All dosages are given as ADULT only. Check your protocols for paediatric dosage rates.

The administration of pharmacological agents by persons other than a qualified medical practitioner, is restricted to incidents in which lawful use is under the authority of the service's medical officer. The authority is vested in the person either through direct consultation or by way of authorised protocols.

THE USE AND POSSESSION OF DRUGS OUTSIDE LAWFUL OPERATIONAL DUTY IS ILLEGAL.

Adrenalin tartrate is a naturally occurring adrenergic stimulant.

Actions

Alpha	—causes peripheral vasoconstriction
Beta-1	—increases the heart rate by increasing the S.A.Node rate
	—increases the conduction velocity through the A.V.Node
	—increases ventricular irritability and the force of myocardial contraction
Beta-2	—causes bronchodilation

Adrenalin tartrate is metabolised by enzymes in the blood, the liver and around nerve endings.

The primary emergency use is in the management of asystole, ventricular fibrillation and anaphylaxis.

Dosage
(1:1000)
0.2-1.0 ml IMI or IVI
Usually given in small increments over a period of time (10 minutes)

Side effects
Tachycardia, ventricular and supraventricular dysrhythmias, hypertension and pupillary dilation

Aminophylline is a smooth muscle relaxant, in particular, of respiratory bronchial smooth muscle.

Actions

Respiratory	—bronchodilation
Cardiac	—a cardiac stimulant, increasing heart rate and cardiac output
	—stimulates vasodilation and diuresis
	—causes anxiety, excitement and restlessness.

Aminophylline is mainly metabolised by the liver.

The primary emergency use is in bronchospasm which does not respond to salbutamol therapy.

Dosage
(250 mg/10 ml)
250-500 mg IVI slow administration over 10 minutes

Side effects
Tachycardia, hypotension, nausea and vomiting, headache and convulsion.

Atropine sulphate is a vagal blocking agent.

Actions

Cardiac   —increases the S.A.Node rate and hence the heart rate

             —increases the conduction velocity through the
              A.V.Node

Atropine is metabolised by the liver.

The primary emergency use is in the management of bradycardia arrythmias.

Dosage

0.4-0.6 mg IMI or IVI

Side effects

Tachycardia, pupillary dilation, dry mouth and blurred vision

Dextrose 50% is a hypertonic crystalloid solution composed of sugar and water.

Action

Provides a ready source of energy.

Dextrose is broken down in most tissues and is stored in the liver as glycogen.

The primary emergency use is in suspected hypoglycaemia.

Dosage

20 ml IVI slowly (initial dose)
50 ml maximum dose

Diazepam is a central nervous system depressant commonly presented as 'Valium'.

Actions

(CNS)   —hypnotic and anti-convulsant

Diazepam is metabolised by the liver.

The primary emergency uses are sedation and anti-convulsant management in status epilepticus and convulsions associated with lignocaine and aminophylline toxicity.

Dosage

2-10 mg IMI or IVI

Side effects

Respiratory depression and hypotension

9

Frusemide is a diuretic agent, commonly seen as 'Lasix'.

Actions
Promotes diuresis
Cardiac   —causes venous dilation and decreases venous return

Frusemide is excreted by the kidneys.
    The primary emergency use is in the management of acute left ventricular failure.

Dosage
20-40 mg IMI or IVI

Side effects
Hypotension.

Glyceryl trinitrate (GTN), commonly seen as 'Anginine', principally acts on vascular smooth muscle as a relaxant.

Actions
Cardiac   —reduces myocardial oxygen demand by arterial and venous dilation
          —reduces blood pressure while usually maintaining coronary perfusion pressure.

GTN is metabolised by the liver.
    The primary emergency use is chest pain of cardiac origin.

Dosage
(600 mcgm tablet)
600 to 900 mcgm

Side effects
Bradycardia, hypotension and headache.

Lignocaine hydrochloride is a ventricular anti-arrythmic drug.

Actions
Cardiac   —depresses the excitability of the myocardium and causes a slight decrease in the conduction velocity of the AV Node.

Lignocaine is principally metabolised by the liver, but a small amount (about 10%) is excreted unchanged by the kidneys.
    The primary emergency use is in ventricular arrythmias and following reversion from VF and VT.

Dosage
50-100 mg IVI

Side effects
Drowsiness, blurred vision, slurred speech, convulsion

Methoxyflurane or 'Penthrane' is an inhalation anaesthetic/analgesic agent.

Action
CNS depressant

The primary emergency use is pain relief in trauma, obstetrics and cardiac disease. However, it is *contraindicated* in patients with severe renal disease and eclampsia.

Dosage
3-6 ml inhalational

Side effects
Altered consciousness

Metoclopramide or 'Maxolon' is an anti-emetic.

Actions
GIT   —accelerates gastric emptying and upper intestinal mobility.

Metoclopramide is metabolised by the liver.
   The primary emergency use is in the management of nausea and vomiting, usually given when administering morphine.

Dosage
(10 mg/2 ml)
0.5 mg/kg bodyweight IMI
May be administered slow IVI

Side effects
Drowsiness, muscle tremor, dry mouth

Morphine sulphate is a narcotic analgesic.

Actions
(CNS)   —depression, producing analgesia
           —depresses respiration and cough reflex
           —stimulates a mood change, pupillary constriction and vomiting
           —addictive

Morphine is metabolised by the liver and excreted by the kidneys.
   The primary emergency use is in pain relief.

Dosage
(10 mg/1 ml or 15 mg/1 ml)
10-20 mg IMI

Side effects
Bradycardia, hypotension, respiratory depression and addiction

9

Naxolone hydrochloride, commonly seen as 'Narcan', is a narcotic antagonist.

Actions
Reverses the effects of narcotics, without causing respiratory depression or pupillary constriction.

Naxolone is metabolised by the liver.
The primary emergency use in the management of respiratory depression associated with narcotic overdose.

Dosage
(0.4 mg/1 ml)
0.4 mg IVI initial dose
Further increments up to maximum 1.2 mg

Side effects
Nausea and vomiting, agitation and convulsion

Salbutamol, commonly seen as 'Ventolin', is synthetic beta-2 agonist.

Action
Causes bronchodilation

Salbutamol is excreted by the kidneys.
The primary use is in the management of respiratory distress associated with acute asthma, smoke inhalation and acute pulmonary oedema.

Dosage
(0.5% solution)
5.0 mg/2.5 ml nebules via aerosol 250 mcgm IVI

Side effects
Tachycardia and muscle tremor

FURTHER READING

Cibulskis M 1982 Essentials of pharmacology. Lippincott, Philadelphia
Opie L et al 1987 Drugs for the heart. Saunders, Philadelphia
Rothenberg M 1987 Advanced medical life support: adult medical emergencies. Mosby, St Louis

SECTION 3
The life cycle

CHAPTER 10
Of birth and children

This chapter explores emergency delivery and the common complications of birth, including the resuscitation of the newborn.

Children are often viewed as 'adults in miniature', a concept which is incorrect. The second part of the chapter describes the uniqueness of children as patients and the approach to managing common paediatric problems.

Topics covered

Normal childbirth
Problems of labour
The paediatric patient
Trauma in children
Child abuse
Poisoning
Paediatric medical emergencies
Sudden infant death

In the course of normal ambulance duties, the ambulance officer is required to deal with sick and injured people, often with tragic outcomes. Therefore it is a unique and joyous experience, albeit rare, to participate in the birth of new life.

10

NORMAL CHILDBIRTH

Aim

To develop an understanding of normal childbirth and develop skills in managing the normal delivery and common complications of childbirth

Learning plan

1. Read the text information
2. Check your understanding using the knowledge check
3. Practice the skills of delivery using an obstetrics manikin
4. Practice resuscitation skills using the skills statements as a guide

The process of childbirth is known as labour and is divided into 3 stages:

- 1st stage—painful and regular uterine contractions. The neck of the womb (cervix) dilates to its 10cm maximum diameter
- 2nd stage—the child is delivered
- 3rd stage—delivery of the placenta and membranes.

Normal pregnancy and labour is a natural process and there is no justification for emergency transport to hospital. Rough handling may adversely affect the mother and newborn.

TO DELIVER OR NOT TO DELIVER

It is important to assess whether there is time to transport the mother-to-be to the nearest hospital capable of managing the birth.

- Has the mother-to-be the uncontrollable urge to push and a desire to open her bowels?
- After discrete inspection of the perineal area, is there evidence of 'crowning' (the appearance of the presenting part, which is normally the scalp) at the vaginal opening?

If the answer to these questions is yes, then there is probably little time left to transport and you are about to assist with a delivery. If the answer is no, then commence transport, but be aware that the birth may occur during the journey, necessitating stopping to assist with the delivery. During transit:

- Reassure the mother-to-be
- Position in a lateral (or Sims) posture
- Administer analgesia during contractions if required
- Maintain routine observations in addition to perineal inspection
- Place the midwifery equipment close by
- Seek a history (if it is the first pregnancy, it may be some time before delivery)
- Notify the hospital to prepare to receive the mother-to-be and newborn.

SECOND STAGE DELIVERY PROCEDURE

Once crowning has commenced, the birth is imminent. Position the mother-to-be supine (on her back), with the knees flexed and the thighs apart. Apply sterile gloves and prepare the equipment, continually observing the perineal area. Place a sterile towel from the kit under the mother's buttocks.

When the next contraction commences, place the mother in the 'bearing-down' posture (Fig. 10.1) and instruct her to 'push'. As the baby's head continues crowning, exert downward pressure (flexion) on the baby's head, with closed fingers. Once the baby's head is delivering, it must not be let go. Instruct the mother to 'pant'. If the membranes are intact over the baby's head, they must be broken carefully.

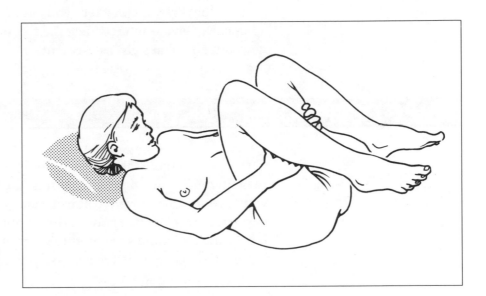

Fig. 10.1 The bearing-down posture to aid delivery of the baby.

Once the baby's face is clear, wipe away any blood or mucous from the mouth and nose in a downward direction. If the mother opens her bowels during the delivery, cover the faeces to prevent contamination of the delivery area. Aspirate the baby's mouth to remove any fluids.

Maintaining control of the baby's head. Check to ensure the umbilical cord is not around the neck. If it is, attempt to slip the cord gently over the head. If the cord is too tightly wrapped around the neck, apply cord clamps and cut in between.

The baby's head will now turn to one side to deliver the shoulders. Place one hand either side of the head with the fingers to the baby's chin. Gently guide the head downwards to assist the delivery of the upper shoulder. A *small* push from mother may be necessary to help the shoulder delivery. Guide the baby's head upward to assist the delivery of the upper shoulder. Support the neck and continue the delivery of the body in an upward direction.

10

Once delivered, place the baby on the mother's abdomen in a head low position. Note the time of the delivery immediately the baby is delivered. Ensure that the baby's airway is clear, using a small oral aspirator gently as required. Check breathing, which is usually established within 1 minute of birth.

The umbilical cord is clamped and cut immediately following the delivery. Use the clamps carried in most midwifery kits (sterile ties are the alternative).

- **Apply one clamp 20 cm away from the baby**
- **Apply a second clamp a further 5 cm along the cord.**

The cord is cut between the clamps and the ends of the cord are swabbed with an antiseptic swab to reduce the possibility of infection. The clamps should be checked to ensure that they are secure and no bleeding is evident.

Now that baby is delivered, you have *2 patients* to care for and it is advisable to give your crewmate the task of completing the care of the newborn and vital signs assessment.

CARE OF MOTHER

Check the mother's abdomen to exclude the presence of a second twin. In most cases of multiple births, the mother already knows and your history taking will confirm such a possibility. Examine the perineal area for tears, applying digital pressure with a pad if bleeding is present. Clean and keep mother warm and dry. Place a pad over the vagina. Complete a vital signs assessment. Collect all blood stained material and take to hospital.

CARE OF NEWBORN

Complete a vital signs assessment. The normal ranges of vital signs for the newborn are as shown in the box.

Normal ranges of newborn vital signs

- Respiratory rate: 30-40 breaths per minute
- Pulse rate: 120-140 beats per minute
- Colour: usually 'pink', although the hands and feet may remain a bluish colour.

A widely used clinical evaluation is the APGAR SCORE. This evaluation should be conducted *1 minute* after delivery and repeated at *5 minutes*. The scoring system (Fig. 10.2) provides a total up to a maximum of 10. The majority of newborns have a satisfactory score within the range of 7-10. A newborn with a score of 4-6 has moderate depression, usually due to poor respiration, necessitating respiratory support. A score below 4 indicates a sick newborn, requiring resuscitation.

APGAR SCORING SYSTEM			
	0 points	**1 point**	**2 points**
Appearance	Blue, pale	body pink, extremities blue	totally pink
Pulse	absent	<100	>100
Grimace	none	grimaces	cries
Activity	limp	flexion of extremities	active motion
Respiratory effort	absent	slow and irregular	good strong cry

Fig. 10.2 The APGAR score.

As soon as possible, the newborn should be dried and wrapped in at least 2 baby blankets to maintain body temperature. Cover the head to reduce heat loss and use the ambulance heater to maintain a warm environment, especially if it is cold.

As soon as convenient, give the mother the baby to nurse, preferably placed to the breast as this will aid uterine contraction.

Transport to hospital can now be resumed. Do not wait for the third stage delivery as this will normally not occur for about 20 minutes after the birth of the baby.

THIRD STAGE DELIVERY

10

The indications of the beginning of the third stage are a small bright blood loss and a lengthening of the cord of about 5 cm. Apply pressure behind the symphysis pubis and if the cord moves back in, the placenta is not yet ready to deliver. If the cord remains steady, check the uterine fundus. It should be contracted and feel firm, about the size of a grapefruit. Attempt to move the uterus gently from side to side. If this can be done, the placenta is ready for delivery.

The placenta is delivered by *controlled* cord traction. However, if you are *unsure* whether the placenta is ready to be delivered, *do not pull on the cord.*

If there is no bleeding evident, there is no indication for the ambulance officer to attempt delivery of the placenta.

Procedure

Place one hand above the symphysis pubis, to displace the uterus downward and prevent it being inverted. Apply *gentle* traction downward on the cord with the other hand. This assists the placenta to descend into the vagina.

When the placenta can be seen, guide the cord upwards and use both hands to cradle the placenta, twisting it around carefully to complete the delivery of the membranes. Once delivered, place the placenta and membranes in a container to be examined at hospital. Note the time of delivery.

The uterine fundus should now be massaged to ensure firm contraction and prevent bleeding. It should feel hard and about the size of a cricket ball.

Make sure mother is clean and dry and check the perineal area again for tears. Routinely check the uterine fundus every 5 minutes and observe for vaginal loss, noting the amount and colour.

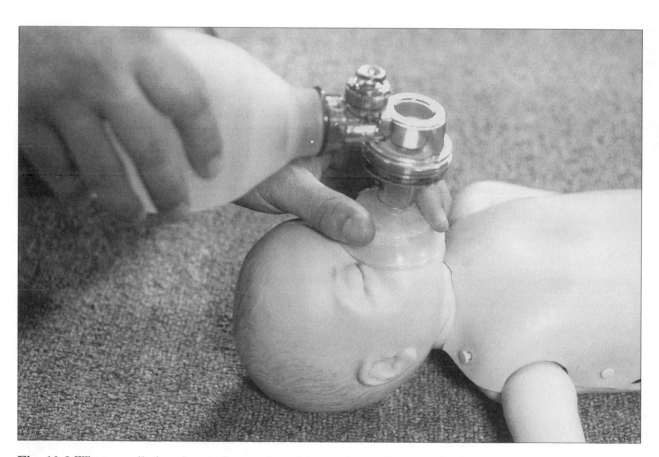

Fig. 10.3 When ventilating the newborn using a bag-mask ventilator, maintain the head in a neutral position.

PROBLEMS OF LABOUR

There are 2 major problems which may present after delivery. The first complication is *maternal bleeding,* commonly due to the failure of the uterus to contract. Excessive bleeding can be life threatening and requires urgent transport to hospital. Uterine fundus massaging will help it to contract. Place the mother in a 'head low' position, with the lower limbs elevated and administer high flow oxygen. Notify the hospital.

The second post-delivery complication is the failure of the new-born to breathe. Check the airway and aspirate if necessary. Apply tactile stimulation (tapping the soles of the feet). If there is no response, commence ventilation with 100% oxygen supplement.

Do not hyperextend the newborn's head.

The head is already in a position of partial flexion and requires only minor extension to open the airway (Fig. 10.3).

The normal ventilation rate is 30-60 breaths per minute. If the pulse is absent, commence CPR, with a compression rate of 100-120 per minute.

TASK Newborn CPR   297

Breech presentation
A newborn delivering other than in the normal head first posture is referred to as a breech presentation. This is usually buttocks and legs first. In such presentations it is best to leave alone and transport to hospital without delay. If the delivery has commenced, support the legs and body until the delivery is complete and continue with normal care, noting the type of presentation for the hospital.

The risk with breech delivery is compression of the umbilical cord by the baby's head in the vaginal canal. If the head is not delivered within 3 minutes the child will suffocate. Using the index and middle finger of one *gloved* hand, gently slide into the vagina in a V formation to pass either side of the baby's nose. Push against the vaginal wall until the head is delivered or the mouth and nose are clear.

IF THE HEAD DOES NOT DELIVER FURTHER, DO NOT PULL

10

Clear the airway and resuscitate if necessary. Transport to hospital immediately with the mothers buttocks and thighs elevated.

Prolapsed cord

This is the presentation of the umbilical cord before the baby. The risk is again compression of the cord by the head in the vaginal canal, causing suffocation. Place the mother in the prone knee-chest position (Fig. 10.4), which will assist in easing the cord compression and administer oxygen. Place a *gloved* hand on the presenting part of baby and push gently to ease the compression of the cord. Transport to hospital without delay, maintaining the hand on the presenting part to prevent delivery. If the delivery is well advanced when you first arrive, resuscitation of the newborn will be required as soon as possible.

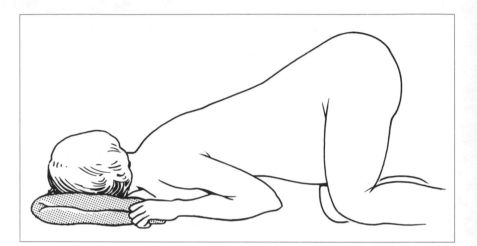

Fig. 10.4 The prone knee-chest position is used to reduce cord compression.

OTHER OBSTETRIC PROBLEMS

Ectopic pregnancy

Fetal development in a fallopian tube, rather than in the uterus, is referred to as ectopic pregnancy. Rupture of the tube will occur as the fetus grows, causing severe bleeding. Transport the patient to hospital immediately, managing the severe abdominal pain with analgesia and administer high flow oxygen.

Eclamptic fits

These fits are the exacerbation of pregnancy toxaemia (eclampsia). This condition is usually pre-diagnosed and the patient is hospitalised during the confinement, as both mother and baby are threatened. Therefore, it is an uncommon incident in pre-hospital care.

The initial clinical picture is one of severe headache with visual disturbance, epigastric pain and vomiting, hypertension and altered consciousness. As the toxaemia develops, convulsion and coma occur, with the risk of cardiac arrest.

Management is urgent transport, with appropriate resuscitation (airway and respiratory support) as necessary.

KNOWLEDGE CHECK

1. What are the 3 stages of labour?

2. Describe the preparation for delivery.

3. Describe the steps in the second stage delivery procedure.

4. What are the normal ranges of vital signs for the newborn?

5. What are the 5 elements of the APGAR score?

6. Describe the steps in the third stage delivery procedure.

7. What is the management for the complication of maternal bleeding following delivery?

8. Describe the management of breech delivery.

9. Describe the management of a prolapsed cord presentation.

10. What does the term ectopic pregnancy mean?

Turn to page 305 to check your answers.

THE PAEDIATRIC PATIENT

Aim

To develop an understanding of children as patients and develop skills in caring for the ill or injured child

Learning plan

1. Read the text information
2. Check your knowledge using the knowledge checks
3. Develop a communication style suitable for dealing with the child patient
4. Practise life support skills using the skills statements as a guide

Children are not only smaller than adults, but are different in structure and function. Consideration of these relative anatomical and physiological differences improves our ability to manage the child in an emergency.

Before considering the differences, we must define paediatric age groups.

- **Newborn—a baby up to the age of 1 month (neonate)**
- **Infant—generally accepted as a baby from 1 month to 2 years**
- **Child (pre-school)—from 2 years to 5 years**
- **Child—generally accepted as 5 years to 12 years. This term is relative and the size of the child must be considered when initiating procedures (CPR).**

10

DIFFERENCES AT A GLANCE

Body proportions. The head is larger, representing 20% of the body area. This is significant when assessing burn injuries.

The airway. The head being larger in a newborn and infant (larger occiput), means that it is already in a position of partial flexion. Opening the airway requires only minor extension.

The jaw is small and the tongue, by proportion, is large. The relatively small oropharynx increases the risk of airway obstruction. A narrow larynx and a large epiglottis increases the risk of obstruction in epiglottitis. The trachea and bronchi are narrow, which means that the effects of mucosal oedema will be evident earlier than in adults.

The thorax. The ribs are horizontal. Therefore respiratory failure risk is greater if the diaphragm is ineffective because of poor chest expansion.

Respiratory function. Breathing is diaphragm dependent. Abdominal pressure may restrict breathing. The breathing rate is higher, therefore artificial ventilation must be at a higher rate. Oxygen utilisation is higher, therefore hypoxia is evident earlier and there is less time to act in an emergency.

Cardiovascular function. The heart rate is faster and blood pressure ranges are lower, therefore cardiac compression rates must be higher. The child has a smaller blood volume, but greater in ratio to body weight than an adult. Therefore the same volume of blood loss in a child than an adult will be more critical. The response to hypoxia and hypotension is often a bradycardia, the opposite to an adult.

Temperature. This tends to rise quickly in disease, peaking rather than a prolonged elevation. The child is prone to febrile convulsions. The relatively large body surface/mass ratio exacerbates heat loss and the child is likely to become rapidly hypothermic.

Fluid balance. The delicate nature of fluid balance, particularly in the newborn and infant, means that they are prone to dehydration.

The immune system. This is less developed and thus the child is susceptible to infection. However, the course of illness tends to be a rapid succumbing and equally rapid recovery.

The ranges of normal physiological values for paediatric patients are essential knowledge when determining the body's response to insult. The accepted ranges per minute at rest are shown in the box.

Normal physiological values of paediatric patients

	Respiratory rate	Pulse rate	BP*
NEWBORN	30–40	120–140	70
INFANT	20–35	80–130	70
CHILD	15–25	70–120	70

(*the blood pressure figure is the accepted *lower* limit of the systolic range only)

Dealing with paediatric patients requires some understanding of their psychological development. The newborn and infant up to about 6 months of age is usually happy being nursed by a parent. At this stage, the child is not frightened by strangers and will normally not object.

The infant up to the age of 2 years tends to dislike being restrained. At this stage, a child is developing the sense of trust and it is important not to frighten him or her. Ask the parent to hold and undress the child if necessary. Children tend to be easily distracted and the infant may be quite happy playing with your torch or keys.

Young pre-schoolers, 2–3 years of age, are probably the most difficult patients. They tend to be negative (saying 'no' to everything) and cling to a parent. They have limited verbal skills but understand reasonably well. The best approach is to do what has to be done as quickly and painlessly as possible.

The 4–5 year old is generally more cooperative and enjoys interacting with adults. Given simple cues, the child is capable of providing a good history.

School age children respond well to being informed about what is happening. They tend to be independent and cooperative, but like privacy, especially for exposure of their bodies. They will generally accept treatment, but still like to have parents around.

Children of the age of 11 or 12 may be developing a greater awareness of their bodies and show the concern of adolescents. They may require privacy during history taking and examination.

Communicating with the child patient is an essential part of management.

- Be calm, confident and patient
- Establish eye contact
- Sit at the level of the child
- Call the child by name
- Do not approach with a lot of equipment. Let the child play with the equipment first if time permits and explain its use
- Talk to the child, not just to the parents
- Do not lead the child. If you ask 'Does it hurt here?'—the answer will probably be yes. The young child cannot describe pain. The severity is best determined by seeking from the parents the effects the pain has had on the child's behaviour. Pain which prevents eating, sleeping and play is usually severe

10

- Use a favourite toy during the examination. You may find the child will tell you where the toy hurts rather than talk about him/ herself
- If possible, examine the problem area last. It is essential to remember that a separated and frightened child will regress in behaviour until returned to a familiar environment or trusting relationship.

KNOWLEDGE CHECK

11. What are the 4 paediatric age groups?

12. Describe the 7 physiological differences between children and adults.

13. What are the ranges of vital signs for each of the paediatric age groups?

14. Describe the essentials of communicating with children.

Turn to page 305 to check your answers.

TRAUMA IN CHILDREN

The newborn has an immature musculoskeletal system. As growth proceeds, the functions of the bones, muscles, tendons and ligaments develop in an integrated manner. During the growth process, their skeletons are more easily damaged by minor twists and falls, resulting in fracture. Sprains and strains are common soft tissue injuries.

Fractures in infancy are usually due to birth trauma, accidents or abuse. Injury in this age group requires further investigation, because apart from road traffic crashes, 'true' accidents rarely occur.

Accidents and trauma are the most common cause of death in children between the ages of 1 and 4 years. These are the inquisitive years, during which parental vigilance is essential. Over recent years, there has been a decrease in childhood deaths, partly attributable to improved government actions; e.g., restraint legislation for motor vehicle passengers, backyard pool fencing legislation and child-proof lids on drug containers.

A child's response to trauma is often rapid and severe complications can occur if adequate intervention is delayed. As with all patients, airway management is *vital*. Inhalation of foreign objects (e.g., buttons, coins, and small pieces of toys) is a frequent emergency in young age groups. (Management strategies were discussed in Chapter 2.)

Blood loss

In children loss of blood is a more serious affair and requires rapid control to conserve the child's smaller volume. Soft tissue injuries, especially to the face and hands, are important and often require plastic surgery repair to damaged nerves and tendons. Lacerations to the scalp may bleed to the extent of significant hypovolaemia and must be controlled by direct pressure early in the management of the patient.

Internal or concealed bleeding may result from falls (bicycles and skateboards) or following crushing by an object or person. The history of the incident is vital in determining the possible internal damage, as often there is little evidence of injury apart from abdominal tenderness.

Head injuries

Injury to the head, especially from falls and impact with a motor vehicle, is potentially serious. The history of the incident is again vital information to help in determining the nature of the injury. Children under 18 months, when the fontanelle is open, may bleed into the skull vault to the extent of producing significant hypovolaemia. This clinical picture of 'shock' in a head injured adult patient would suggest blood loss in other locations rather than from the head injury.

Convulsion due to cerebral hypoxia may result and management must be directed towards effective airway support and adequate oxygenation. Maintain observations of vital signs and transport to the emergency department without delay.

Facial injury

An injury to the face may result in damage to the teeth. A tooth that has been completely removed can be replaced provided it is kept moist and the delay between insult and hospital intervention is not long. The mouth should be examined carefully because often what appears to be a tooth completely knocked out can be one which has been impacted into the gums.

Eye injury

It is difficult to examine eye injuries as children will generally not permit a good look at their eyes. If the injury does not involve chemical splash, cover both eyes and transport in a sitting posture to the emergency department. However, if the injury is a result of chemical splash, the eyes *must* be irrigated with copious fluid (water or saline eye wash) and continued until arrival at the emergency department.

Fractures

In children fractures tend to be stable, with often only slight displacement. Cervical spinal injury is rare before the teenage years, but may occur in diseased bone. Upper limb fractures are the most common

10

and those affecting the wrist and elbow should be carefully examined and observed for disruption to blood flow. Oxygen therapy, especially in long bone fractures, will reduce the tendency towards fatty embolus development, a potential complication in children.

Immobilisation of fractures can be achieved more simply than in adult patients. Anatomical splinting (tying the legs together) or the use of a pillow as a splint is normally the most effective approach. Immobilisation reduces pain, but analgesia may be necessary. However, parental consent should be obtained before administration. Young children are often difficult patients to give analgesia to because of their fear of masks.

Burn injuries

In young children, burn injuries, especially moist burns (scalds) are common. Flame burns tend to occur in older age groups. Regardless of this differentiation, burn injuries form a large percentage of emergency admissions to hospitals. The assessment of burns in children requires a modification to that used for adult patients, because of the

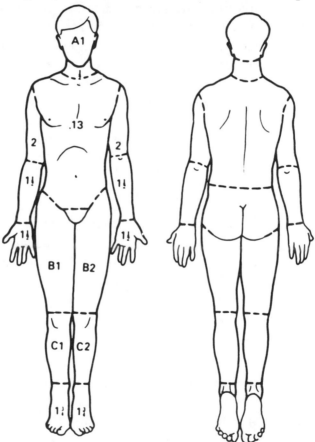

Fig. 10.5 The Lund and Browder method for assessing the surface area of burns especially in children. (Reproduced with permission from Chandler J 1991 Tabbner's nursing care: theory and practice, 2nd edition. Churchill Livingstone, Melbourne)

Body proportions (percentages) affected by growth

	0	1	5	10	15	Adult age
A half head	9.5	8.5	6.5	5.5	4.5	3.5
B half one thigh	2.75	3.25	4	4.25	4.5	4.75
C half one leg	2.5	2.5	2.75	3	3.25	3.5

To estimate the total of the body surface area burned, the percentages assigned to the burned areas are added. The total is then an estimate of the burn size.

proportion differences (discussed earlier in this chapter). A guide to area assessment is the Lund and Browder chart (Fig. 10.5). A useful 'rule of thumb' is the area of the patient's palm and fingers, which is about 1%. A burn area of 10% or more in a child is a serious injury and requires urgent care and transport to the emergency department.

Drowning

Deaths from drowning and the effects of immersion are a frequent event, especially during the summer months. Laryngospasm normally prevents the inhalation of large volumes of water and the prognosis is usually good if resuscitation is commenced early at the scene. Immersion in cold water reduces the body's core temperature and this hypothermic state tends to prolong the time interval between clinical and biological death. Resuscitation attempts should continue until medical intervention advises otherwise, as good survival has been achieved even following long periods of immersion.

CHILD ABUSE

Non-accidental trauma results in about 1 in 20 hospital trauma admissions a year. Child protection agencies deal annually with thousands of children who are physically, emotionally, or sexually abused.

Studies indicate that there is no distinction between socioeconomic groups, but the majority of parents involved come from an unhappy environment, often related to depression and criminal records. Interference with the bonding process between mother and infant may also lead to child abuse. The majority of abused children exhibit delay in speech development and frequently fail in academic pursuits.

The ambulance officer plays an important role in recording and reporting the nature of the incident to the medical officer. However, it is *not* the officer's province to *judge* the people involved. Noting of history, patterns of injury and the stories provided are the extent of the task, along with appropriate patient care for the victim. Some of the features to be aware of and note are:

- Injuries which are not consistent with the parent's story—e.g., the parent may claim that the child fell into a hot bath, yet the buttocks are the only area burned
- Injuries which are inconsistent with the child's motor development—parents may claim that the child (especially young infants) was injured through adventure, when it is obvious that the child could not have achieved such activity
- Injuries at variant stages of resolution—e.g., a mixture of old and new bruising and grazes
- The parent's story is often vague
- The parent's demeanour is often unusual—often the mother is also abused. Itinerant behaviour and unemployment, single parent families and other social pressures are often evident.

10

POISONING

The most common form of poisoning in children is ingestion of substances, especially medicines and substances found in any household—e.g., soap powders, carpet shampoo, window cleaning fluids, deodorant blocks.

Paracetamol is a common poison in children, with a toxic dose of 210 mg/kg—i.e., more than 5 tablets (of 500 mg strength) are toxic for a 2-year-old. The drug causes gastric irritation, evidenced by abdominal pain, nausea and vomiting and anorexia, usually within 2-14 hours following ingestion. Ingestion of a toxic level of paracetamol may cause liver damage and jaundice, which may not be evident for several days. Therefore, it is essential for the patient to be hospitalised. Immediate care requires emesis with Syrup of Ipecac.

Iron (ferrous gluconate, ferrous sulphate, ferrogradumet) is another commonly ingested poison. More than 200 mg of elemental iron is toxic to a 2 year old child (e.g., 6 ferrous gluconate 300 mg tablets, or 2 ferrogradumet 350 mg tablets). Gastric irritation (abdominal pain, vomiting and diarrhoea) is an early sign of poisoning, occurring usually within 2 hours following ingestion. Toxicity is evidenced by tachycardia, hypotension, pallor and cyanosis. The child may appear quite well initially, but sudden circulatory collapse may occur. Emesis with Syrup of Ipecac is again the first order treatment; transport to the emergency department without delay.

Deodorant blocks will cause toxicity in children if the amount ingested is more than 20 gm. Emesis should again be used as the first order treatment. If the wrapper is still available, check for first aid instructions, because some of these substances react with water or milk. If there is some doubt about the action of the substance, contact the Poisons Information Centre for advice.

Corrosive and irritant substances (e.g., dish washer detergents, pool chlorine granules and petroleum products) must not be managed by inducing vomiting. This may cause further tissue damage and risk inhalation of fumes into the airway and lungs. Milk or other fluids may help to reduce gastric irritation if the child will accept them. Transport to the emergency department without delay.

PAEDIATRIC MEDICAL EMERGENCIES

During the years of growth and development, the child succumbs to a variety of infections and common diseases, which provide little or no threat. However, there are 4 events which frequently require ambulance intervention and hospitalisation.

Croup

A respiratory problem, croup commonly occurs in the age range of 2–4 years. Normally, the cause is a viral infection of the upper respiratory tract. The significant feature is the characteristic harsh 'croupy' cough, with an inspiratory stridor (whistling sound). The symptoms tend to be worse at night, especially during cold periods. In most cases, the parents have usually commenced treatment with a croupette vaporiser or placed the child in a steamy bathroom to improve respiratory flow. This should be continued for 10–20 minutes, maintaining reassurance and observation of vital signs. The child should be transported to the emergency department in a warm environment. Use the heater in the vehicle especially if it is cold, and transport quietly to hospital.

Epiglottitis

Epiglottitis is a more serious airway problem of acute onset, usually due to bacterial infection. Commonly occurring in the age range of 1–4 years, epiglottitis is inflammation of the tissues above the vocal cords. This inflammation may occlude the airway and is potentially fatal. The significant features are a sore throat and inability to swallow. Stridor may be evident in some cases. The patient tends to sit forward and looks anxious and sick out of proportion to obstruction. Transport the patient immediately to the emergency department in a sitting posture. Caution should be exercised with the use of warning devices as this may distress the patient and exacerbate the problem. *Do not examine* the throat as this may antagonise the tissues further. Oxygen therapy should be commenced, preferably via a humidifier. Observation of vital signs, with particular attention to the airway and respiratory function, should be maintained frequently. Be alert to the possibility of total airway obstruction.

Febrile convulsions

High, untreated fever is often the cause of febrile convulsions. In the very young infant (up to 6 months), the cause may be due to the immaturity of sweating and temperature control mechanisms. Febrile convulsions tend to peak at about 2 years and cease after about the 7 year age, although uncontrolled and sustained high temperatures (hyperpyrexia) may cause convulsion in older patients.

10

The seizure tends to be of a self-limiting nature with a short episode of body twitching, rolling of the eyes and accompanied by frothy salivation. Following the seizure, the child may be drowsy and confused. Cyanosis is often evident during the seizure, but normal colour returns quickly.

The aim of immediate management is to reduce the temperature. Frequently, the child is wearing too many clothes, which retain body heat, or is being nursed by the parent, which transfers body heat. Remove the clothing and cool the skin by sponging with tepid water. However, care should be taken not to induce shivering, as this is the body's natural mechanism to conserve heat. The patient should be transported to the emergency department quietly for observation and management of the cause.

Dehydration

The fourth problem of significance is dehydration. Commonly gastroenteritis and hot weather are the causes of dehydration in young children. The greater body surface area to weight ratio, proportionately larger gastrointestinal tract and higher metabolic rate tends to exacerbate body fluid loss. Burn injury is another cause of rapid dehydration in young children.

Tachycardia and dry mucous membranes are significant features, along with increased body temperature and decreased urine output. The patient should be transported to the emergency department, maintaining a comfortable environment in the vehicle. Oxygen administration is indicated in cases of increased respiratory rate or altered consciousness.

KNOWLEDGE CHECK

15. What are the 5 features to be aware of when dealing with child abuse?

16. What is meant by the term emesis?

17. Describe the management of a patient with non-corrosive poisoning.

18. Describe the management of a patient with corrosive poisoning.

19. What is the significant feature of croup?

20. Describe the management of epiglottitis.

Turn to page 306 to check your answers.

SUDDEN INFANT DEATH SYNDROME (SIDS)

SIDS or cot death is 'sudden death of any infant or child which is unexpected by history and in which a thorough post-mortem examination fails to demonstrate an adequate cause of death' (2nd International Conference on Causes of SIDS, Seattle, USA, 1969). Currently, the death rate world wide is of the order of 2 infants per 1000 births.

Commonly, children in the age range of 2-5 months are affected, but SIDS may also occur in both younger and older infants. There are several features associated with cot death, which create special problems for the grieving parents and should be recognised by the ambulance officer:

- The parents have no time to prepare for their loss because of the sudden and unexpected nature of the event.
- The impact on the parents, especially the mother, is great because it is usually during the time when bonding is intense.
- The absence of reason for the death produces deep anxiety.
- Parents experience feelings of guilt, blaming themselves for the child's death.
- The police investigation, while routine by law, tends to reinforce guilt feelings and uncertainty.

The ambulance crew responding to a cot death should attempt some form of resuscitation. While parents know that the child is dead, the fact that something is attempted by the crew is appreciated. Support for the parents is the vital task for the ambulance officer. Do not separate them from the child. Allow them to hold the child if they desire. Explaining that you believe it is a cot death and that nothing could have been done to save the child will help to minimise guilt feelings.

Explain to the parents that the police will call and that this is a routine investigation in all cases of sudden death. It is important to reinforce the fact that there is no suspicion that it is the parents' fault. Sit with them and allow them to grieve, but inform them of what is to happen. Include the parents in the decision making about where the child is to be taken and who to notify. Offer to contact family, friends or a minister of religion.

The SIDS Foundation can be contacted 24 hours a day and provides a counsellor to assist the parents.

10

FURTHER READING

Guntheroth W 1982 Crib death: the sudden infant death syndrome. Futura, New York

Lord J D, 1987 When a baby dies. Hill of Content, Melbourne

Miller A W F, Callander R 1989 Obstetrics Illustrated, 4th edn. Churchill Livingstone, Edinburgh

Robinson M J, 1990 Practical Paediatrics, 2nd edn. Churchill Livingstone, Melbourne

Wren B, Lobo R 1989 Handbook of obstetrics and gynaecology. Chapman Hill, London

CHAPTER 11
Of ageing

As we get older, and progress from the nursery to the nursing home, we undergo physical and mental changes. The degeneration of our bodies and minds gives rise to disease and dysfunction and we become more frequent users of the health care system. This chapter explores the ageing process and the problems of ageing.

Topics covered

The age continuum
Physical dysfunction
Mental dysfunction

All the world's a stage,
and all the men and women merely players.
They have their exits and their entrances,
And one man in his time plays many parts,
His act being seven ages...

Shakespeare, *As You Like It*

THE AGE CONTINUUM

Aim

To develop an understanding of the ageing process and the needs of the elderly patient

Learning plan

1. Read the text information
2. Do an investigation of your own family and identify the needs of each age group

11

The study of the age continuum extends Shakespeare's seven ages to nine age ranges by the inclusion of:

• In utero—from conception to birth
• Newborn—from birth to one month.

Human development is dramatic during the first two decades of life. But the next five to six decades are equally as complex and important for the individual, for those around them and for those who advise and provide health care. In the previous chapter, the focus was the early years from birth, through infancy and childhood, so let's pick up the continuum from adolescence.

Adolescence (12-18 years)

The teenage years are generally a healthy period of life, but motor car crashes, alcohol and drugs take their toll. Adolescents are preoccupied with the physical changes occurring in their bodies and the influence of peer groups. This period is often the beginning of rebellion—the conflict between parental control and freedom.

Biological changes herald puberty (and in the female, the menarche) and lead to sexual activity. However, the adolescent is frequently moody during this period of great change and the female is vulnerable to the 'slimmer's disease' (anorexia nervosa). Depression and suicide start to occur and schizophrenia has been identified as a major mental illness in the late teen years.

The young adult (18-30 years)

This is probably the healthiest age of the continuum. Physical growth stops and we reach the peak of strength. We achieve emotional independence and generally have an optimistic view of the world around us, with a place in society and starting our own family. However, many young adults suffer stresses and depression related to financial planning and career choices.

Motor car crashes and sporting injuries are the common causes of physical distress, and may lead to mental health problems now that the young adult has responsibilities. Pregnancy and contraception are often a problem for the young woman.

The prime of life (30-42 years)

Generally, the prime of life is the most stable period of our lives. We are established in both a career and a home. However, it is often the time of greatest financial stress, with children at school and a mortgage to pay. Some people go through a period of disillusionment, which is referred to as the mid-life crisis.

Physically, it is the time where a slight decrease occurs and the problems of high blood pressure begin to emerge. Chronic bronchitis, lung cancer and breast cancers are becoming more common. However, motor car crashes are still the major cause of death in this age group.

Middle age (42-60 years)

This is generally the period of contentment. The family has grown and grandchildren are the expectation. However, this is also the age of marriage breakdown and work redundancy. Physically, the body is slowing down and there is a noticeable decrease in stature and strength. Menopause occurs in women.

Degenerative disease processes emerge as a significant problem in this age group. Cancers, particularly of the bowel and breast, together with cardiovascular disease are the most common problems.

Old age (60 years and over)

Physically, the body is now tiring and we are no longer capable of maintaining the degree of activity of our earlier years. The focus is now on ourselves and coming to terms with retirement.

It is often the period of life where loneliness becomes a factor, with the loss of loved-ones and separation from family members. Memory failure and a tendency for reduced communication exacerbate the feelings of loneliness.

Problems of cardiovascular disease and cancers are common. Arthritis limits mobility and we become more dependent on the health system. Senility does not affect every person, but dementia is seen in this age group.

PHYSICAL DYSFUNCTION

Heredity seems to have some bearing on our life span and is probably predetermined from the time of conception. An expectation of living for a period similar to our parents is therefore quite realistic.

People age physically at differing rates. Cardiovascular degeneration, in particular atherosclerosis, is more prevalent in Western society than in under developed countries. As the disease progresses, hypertension and a decrease in tissue perfusion occurs. The arteries lose their ability to constrict (a reflex mechanism in compensating for changes in homeostasis) and hence, significant hypotension may occur in emergency situations.

The myocardium becomes less compliant as fibrous tissue replaces heart muscle, resulting in reduced ability to increase cardiac output, again causing profound hypotension. Poor tissue perfusion is most commonly seen peripherally, where the skin becomes thin and shows a tendency to peel, crack and ulcerate easily. Peripheral blood vessels are damaged by minimal trauma, often resulting in large bruised areas of skin.

Degeneration of the bony framework is commonly seen in two forms, osteomalacia and osteoporosis.

11

Osteomalacia is softening of bone. Although it is not normally a feature of ageing directly (it is seen in children and goes by the common name of rickets), it signifies other pathological disorder. This is usually vitamin D deficiency through poor diet and problems of absorption and activation of the vitamin, due to bowel, liver and renal disease. The elderly patient is therefore predisposed to fracture, frequently seen as fractures of the shaft and neck of femur.

Osteoporosis is a reduction in the total amount of bone mass, due to a reduction of both protein and mineral fractions of the bone. Minimal forces may result in multiple fracture and is commonly seen in fractures of the neck of femur and vertebrae. Although the cause is largely unknown, immobility, poor diet and lack of circulating oestrogens (in the elderly female) are predisposing factors.

Ageing processes affect the brain. A reduction in brain cells and thinning of grey matter results in a decrease of the total brain weight. However, this does not necessarily mean there is an associated deterioration in mental capacity. Peripheral nerves change subtly, causing loss of fine sensation, position sense and temperature and pain sensation. The changes in pain perception may result in an elderly patient not being aware of the pain of a fracture; rather, the person may complain of immobility or, in the case of femur fracture, difficulty walking.

MENTAL DYSFUNCTION

Confusion states commonly accompany emergency and acute situations in the elderly patient. These mental disturbances are called *Acute Brain Syndrome*. However, the disturbance usually subsides once the underlying medical problem is treated (e.g., metabolic, cardiovascular or cerebrovascular disturbances). The association with acute illness is disturbance to homeostasis, in particular acidosis, which is prone to develop in the elderly patient.

The patient presents irritable and agitated, sometimes aggressive and may behave antisocially. Commonly, the span of attention is markedly reduced and the patient seems disoriented and confused. Mis-identification of persons is a frequent disorder of perception and occasionally delusions and hallucinations are seen.

Chronic Brain Syndrome develops slowly and is commonly seen as senile dementia. It affects people in their seventies and eighties and is more common in females. Arteriosclerotic dementia, although less common, may be seen in a slightly younger age range and often follows a CVA.

Behaviour disturbance in both groups presents as apathy, gross memory loss (especially recent memory), disorientation and often marked intellectual loss. Wandering behaviour frequently results in these people being involved in traffic accidents and losing their way, with little ability to advise others of where they belong.

Dementia in younger people (early forties) is known as Alzheimer's Disease and is usually inherited rather than associated with the normal ageing processes.

The distressed elderly patient is a frequent case encountered by the ambulance officer. The approach should be one of considering more than just the medical problem. Note the patient's surroundings, whether they live alone or there is some supervision. Check to see if there is food in the house and whether the place is clean—is the patient clean and dressed? Check for medications and take them with the patient to the hospital. Communication may be difficult and a check for visual or hearing deficit may help you overcome problems and manage the patient more successfully.

The elderly patient is often challenging and demanding. Recognition of the patient as a total entity and not just a clinical problem will result in effective management and a rewarding experience.

FURTHER READING

Blazer D 1982 Depression in later life. Mosby, St Louis
Shaw M 1991 The challenge of ageing: a multidisciplinary approach to extended care, 2nd edn. Churchill Livingstone, Melbourne

11

CHAPTER 12
Of death and dying

While the role of pre-hospital care is aimed towards preventing death, it is not always possible to resuscitate patients. Much of the task is routine health transport, but from time to time, emergency responses to trauma and acute illness inevitably expose the ambulance officer to death and dying.

Understanding the topic of death and importantly, the grieving process, is an essential part of any study of health care.

Topics covered

The grieving process
The dying child

Aim

To develop an understanding of grief process and the empathy necessary in dealing with the dying patient

Learning plan

1. **Read the text information**
2. **Supplement reading with the further reading references given.**

The ambulance officer's role in the provision of pre-hospital patient care involves both health transport and emergency responses. Inevitably, some patients will die in the ambulance or be dead at the scene of an incident. Some will die in a peaceful setting, while others will be found dead in more horrific circumstances.

Chapter 1 provided strategies for coping with crises, but it is important to also understand the grief process, through which patients and relatives must go in order to cope with their loss.

Before the advent of sophisticated medical services, people died usually at home and families generally were familiar with this inevitable event. Today, in a modern society, we are largely divorced from death. Apart from the sudden, unexpected deaths from road crashes and 'collapse', death is viewed as something which happens normally in the hospital or old-folks home. We are exposed through the media

12

to death, but in a sense, deny that such things will happen in our community and certainly not to us. From time to time this denial is shaken by events close to home, but we soon overcome the emotional impact and continue with life's pursuits.

This, of course, is not a bad response. It might be argued that life is too short to be concerned with such morbid events as death and dying. However, health providers and emergency service personnel are not quite so insulated from the reality.

When you look at the 'ages of man', death is the final stage of the growth continuum and is equally important as birth. It is the stage of reconciling achievements and preparing to lose all worldly possessions. The process is one of coming to terms with and accepting one's own finiteness. However, acceptance, the final step in the grief process (Fig. 12.1) may not be reached by all people.

THE GRIEVING PROCESS

A 'normal' healthy state of life is one of stability. As we age, our bodies degenerate and our physical prowess diminishes. We adapt our lifestyle accordingly and cope with most illness and disability. However, terminal illness may manifest at any age in the life continuum, starting the process of grief.

The first stage is usually *denial*. This is the natural tendency in crises to avoid the reality of the situation. A second opinion might be sought in the hope that some mistake has been made in diagnosing the terminal illness. The patient has feelings of loneliness and guilt.

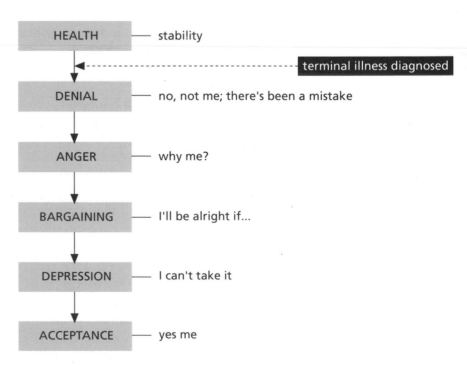

Fig. 12.1 The grief process.
(Adapted from Kubler-Ross E, Death: the final stage of growth.)

Denial gives way to the realisation that 'yes it is me, but why?'. The *anger* is usually self-directed in an attempt to rationalise past actions which might have contributed to the event. However, the anger may be directed towards those around the patient and it is important that this behaviour be tolerated. Remember that the patient is trying to come to terms with the loss of *everything*.

The realisation of 'yes it is me, but why?' turns to the stage of *bargaining* This is the search for alternatives for survival. The patient attempts to find some hope that if medication is taken and treatment is followed correctly, they might yet live. Some patients turn to spiritual beliefs for hope.

The realisation that there is no means by which the inevitable might be avoided causes the stage of *depression*. The patient is often tired of having treatment and may be quite withdrawn. This is a difficult stage for both the patient, the family and health providers.

The final stage is *acceptance*. The patient has now come to terms with the inevitability of their death and can usually talk about it. Many patients find comfort in spiritual beliefs.

It is important to realise that not all patients will arrive at acceptance. It could be said that we live and die 'in character' and thus our passage through the grieving process will stop at an individual stage. Recognition of the stages of grief, then, will help the ambulance officer empathise with the patient during transport to and from hospital.

The family and relatives of the dying patient must also come to terms with the inevitable. The same empathy and care should be exercised to help them cope.

In multicultural societies, it is important to understand that different cultures have differing needs in times of terminal illness and death. For example, Muslims prefer that the dying and deceased should be turned towards Mecca. Death is seen as something predestined by God and they may appear quite calm and accepting. It is important for them to recite the Koran or pray in front of, or near to their loved one. Many Muslims will be conscious of offending the ambulance crew or may conceal their wishes to avoid embarrassment. Handling the body of the deceased should be as little as possible and preferably by a person of the same sex. Muslims believe that pain and pressure can be felt by the deceased and that the soul remains close until burial.

Allowing time where possible and observing cultural differences and needs will maintain the vital elements of empathy and care when dealing with the dying and death event.

12

THE DYING CHILD

The death of a child is extremely difficult to face, because the end of this life is premature and without fulfilment. A child's concept of death is greatly influenced by the attitudes and explanations offered by adults. When death is expected, there is time for anticipatory grieving for the family and time to help the child cope with the fatal prognosis. Children usually adapt to the eventuality of death more quickly than adults. Although they may know that their death is imminent, they may not have been told.

The care of a terminally ill child during transport should be aimed at maintaining a confident and empathetic attitude, rather than one of gloom and doom. Parents should be encouraged to travel with the child.

Sudden death

Sudden death presents the ambulance officer with the problem of dealing with relatives, rather than the patient. Often the parents berate themselves for not preventing the accident or express guilt feelings and remorse for not doing something extra or different with the child.

The sudden death of an adult will give rise to similar feelings of remorse. Take the time to help the family with the necessary arrangements. Be cautious about sharing your own theories with grief-stricken parents or relatives. This may heighten, unwittingly, their guilt feelings. A confident, compassionate approach is the most important role.

FURTHER READING

Abdalati H 1975 Islam in focus. American Trust Publications, Indianapolis

Hinton J 1979 Dying. Penguin, Middlesex

Kubler-Ross E 1982 Living with death and dying. Souvenir Press, London

O'Connor N 1984 Letting go with love: the grieving process. La Mariposa Press, Tucson

APPENDIX A
Practical skills guides

The skills statements in this section are guides to practice and are task specific rather than protocols. Each describes a specific procedure. The management of a patient problem will involve several of these procedures, which may require modification, depending on circumstances.

However, these skills provide the basis for practice and establish the essential framework upon which pre-hospital patient care can be built.

GUIDES LISTED

FORE-AND-AFT LIFT

Equipment	Stages	Key points
Patient Assistant Stretcher	1. Prepare patient.	1. Reassure and inform. 2. Keep covered with blanket or sheet. 3. Instruct patient not to help to ensure safe lifting for both patient and crew.
	2. Prepare stretcher.	1. Place close to patient to reduce carry distance. 2. Lower side rails if applicable. 3. Elevate to the appropriate height if applicable.
	3. Prepare to lift the patient:	1. Sit patient up. 2. Rescuer A: Support behind patient and reach under arms to grasp the forearms and place across the patient's chest. 3. Rescuer B: Squat alongside the patient. Grasp under the knees and small of patient's back.
	4. Lift the patient.	1. Rescuer A takes the weight to balance the lift. 2. Both rescuers lift together slowly. 3. Avoid bending and twisting movements to prevent back injury.
	5. Carry patient to the stretcher.	1. Move slowly and together. 2. Keep the load close to your body to reduce strain.

Notes

This procedure may be contraindicated with patients who have altered consciousness, chest, upper limb and abdominal wall injuries.

PLACING A PATIENT ON A STRETCHER

A

Equipment	Stages	Key points
Ambulance stretcher Patient Assistant	1. Prepare stretcher.	1. Ensure straps or harness are clear. 2. Appropriate height if applicable. 3. Rails down if applicable.
	2. Lift and carry patient.	1. Refer previous skill statement—(fore-and-aft lift). 2. Appropriate to the patient's condition.
	3. Lower patient to stretcher.	1. Lower slowly and together to avoid injury. 2. Support patient's head and shoulders.
	4. Position patient.	1. Appropriate to the condition of the patient. 2. Ensure patient comfort.
	5. Secure patient.	1. Apply stretcher harness or straps.

Notes

Prevent back injury by working together. Bend your knees and keep your back straight.

LOADING A STRETCHER INTO AN AMBULANCE

Equipment	Stages	Key points
Stretcher (trolley type) Ambulance Assistant	1. Prepare stretcher trolley for loading.	1. Adjust to appropriate height for loading. 2. Raise slowly to prevent rescuer injury and patient discomfort.
	2. Position stretcher near open rear of ambulance.	1. Place head end of stretcher close to rear step of the ambulance.
	3. Prepare to load stretcher into the ambulance.	1. Rescuers either side of stretcher at head end.
	4. Load stretcher into ambulance.	1. Lift head end of stretcher onto the floor of the ambulance. 2. If vehicle height requires trolley to be collapsed—one rescuer supports the stretcher while the other activates release mechanism. 3. Slide stretcher into ambulance slowly.
	5. Secure stretcher in ambulance.	1. Locate stretcher in correct position. 2. Engage locking devices.

Unloading procedure
1. Disengage locking devices.
2. Slide stretcher to rear of compartment.
3. Rescuers grasp either side of stretcher and slowly remove from ambulance.
4. Trolley mechanism is activated if applicable.
5. Lower stretcher to ground level.

Notes

If the procedure is performed with a patient, explain what is to happen before commencing.

MOVING A PATIENT USING A CARRY CHAIR

A

Equipment	Stages	Key points
Patient Stretcher/carry chair Assistant	1. Prepare carry chair.	1. Fold stretcher to carry chair configuration. 2. Ensure straps are open. 3. Ensure chair is locked into configuration. 4. Ensure lower carry handles are folded.
	2. Prepare patient.	1. Reassure and inform.
	3. Lift patient to carry chair.	1. Fore-and-aft lift. 2. Secure patient with straps.
	4. Move patient.	1. Ensure patient's arms secure to prevent clutching especially if negotiating stairs. 2. Tilt carry chair to allow wheeling. 3. Move slowly to minimise patient discomfort.

Notes

If negotiating stairs, lift the carry chair by carry handles and descend feet first carefully. Before loading into the ambulance, re-configure the carry chair into the standard stretcher:

- release straps.
- disengage locking devices.
- slide carry chair components slowly into flat position and lock.
- adjust head rest position to patient comfort.
- secure straps.
- load stretcher on to trolley and lock into position.

LIFTING A PATIENT WITH A LIFTING FRAME (JORDON MULTI-LIFT)

Equipment

Patient
Lifting frame
Assistant
Stretcher

Stages	Key points
1. Prepare patient.	1. Ensure no obstacles under patient. 2. Arms against body. 3. Legs straight and together.
2. Position frame.	1. Place carefully over patient. 2. Align top lug with patient's ear.
3. Place and secure gliders.	1. Pass tapered end of gliders under the patient and secure to lugs. 2. Broad glider at patient's head. 3. Adjust tension as required.
4. Position stretcher.	1. Close to patient. 2. Side rails down and harness or straps open. 3. Remove pillow.
5. Lift patient with frame.	1. Rescuers either end of frame. 2. Lift together slowly to prevent injury and patient discomfort.
6. Place frame on stretcher.	1. Lower carefully on to stretcher. 2. Position evenly on stretcher.
7. Secure patient.	1. Cover patient with a blanket. 2. Secure stretcher straps or harness.

Notes

Gliders can be secured to the lugs if required by looping a conforming bandage around each lug. However, the frame is primarily a lifting device and not designed for use as a stretcher. If the patient is longer than the frame, ensure the frame is above the head and allow the heels to extend beyond the frame.

MANUAL AIRWAY CLEARANCE

Equipment	Stages	Key points
Manikin/patient	1. Position patient.	1. Side position to utilise gravity.
	2. Check mouth.	1. Open and look. 2. Remove foreign matter using two 'hooked' fingers in a sweeping action. 3. If dentures are dislodged or loose, remove.
	3. Position patient's head.	1. Tilt head and support jaw. 2. Jaw thrust may be necessary if airway cannot be maintained.
	4. Check breathing.	1. Look for chest/abdomen movement. 2. Listen for air movement. 3. Feel for movement with one hand on chest/abdomen at costal margins.

Notes

If there is no evidence of fluids in the mouth, the patient may be left supine and turn the head to one side for 'finger sweeping'.

Jaw thrust:

Place one hand on each side of the patient's head:

- 5th, 4th and 3rd fingers around the angle of the mandible
- index fingers on the body of the mandible
- thumbs over the zygomas.

Protract the jaw:

at right angles to the line of the pharynx by pressure at the angles of the mandible.

APPLICATION OF SUCTION

Equipment	Stages	Key points
Suction source Catheter Manikin	1. Prepare equipment.	1. Position suction unit conveniently. 2. Select appropriate suction catheter. 3. Attach catheter to suction tubing.
	2. Introduce catheter into patient's mouth.	1. Turn on suction control. 2. Open patient's mouth. 3. Insert catheter in lower corner of the patient's mouth.
	3. Apply suction.	1. Occlude catheter control hole. 2. Sweep across the mouth. 3. Withdraw catheter. 4. Repeat as required. 5. Flush line with water to keep the catheter patent.
	4. Check.	1. Airway clear. 2. Maintain patient's posture.

Notes

Oxygen-powered systems may quickly deplete oxygen reserves. Turn off suction immediately after use. Wide bore suction catheters are preferable in the mobile environment. Care must be taken if a rigid sucker is used.

INSERTION OF AN OROPHARYNGEAL AIRWAY

Equipment	Stages	Key points
Oropharyngeal airway Manikin	1. Check patient's conscious level.	1. Check response. 2. Check for gag reflex.
	2. Prepare OP airway.	1. Select appropriate size. 2. Lubricate with water or patient's saliva.
	3. Insert OP airway.	1. Hold by the flange. 2. Natural curve upside down. 3. Pass tip first and insert halfway into the patient's mouth. 4. Rotate airway 180° while continuing insertion. 5. Insert until the flange rests against patient's lips. 6. Ensure the lower lip is not pinched between the teeth and OP airway.
	4. Check.	1. Check for gag reflex and remove airway at first sign of retching. 2. Maintain position of the airway. 3. Look, listen and feel for air movement.

Notes

The correct size OP airway is essential to afford optimal airway support. If it is too small, the tongue will not be held forward adequately. Too large a size OP airway may cause damage to the mucosa of the oropharynx. Suction equipment should be available for use to remove fluids as necessary.

POSITIONING A PATIENT—LATERAL POSITION

Equipment	Stages	Key points
Patient	1. Position self.	1. Preferred side. 2. Kneel at patient's hips.
	2. Prepare patient.	1. Remove bulky objects from the patient's pockets. 2. Place patient's far arm out straight from shoulder. 3. Fold near arm across chest. 4. Flex near leg at the knee.
	3. Turn patient on side.	1. Grasp at hips and shoulder. 2. Rotate the patient away from you.
	4. Position patient.	1. Draw upper leg towards the head so the knee is flexed at right angles. 2. Flex far arm to bring the hand under the patient's head. 3. Place upper arm flexed by the side of the patient's head, clear of the face.
	5. Check.	1. Firm posture. 2. Check airway and breathing.

Notes

The lateral position is the most easily achieved posture as it utilises the patient's body weight during the turn. Before deciding on the turning method, check which side the patient will be facing when loaded into the ambulance. You may find it difficult to manage a patient who is facing away from you.

POSITIONING A PATIENT—COMA POSITION

Equipment	Stages	Key points
Patient	1. Position self.	1. Preferred side. 2. Kneel at patient's hips.
	2. Prepare patient.	1. Remove bulky objects from the patient's pockets. 2. Place patient's near arm under the buttocks, palm of the hand down. 3. Cross far leg over near leg at ankles. 4. Flex far arm across patient's chest.
	3. Turn patient on side.	1. Grasp far hip. 2. Support patient's head. 3. Rotate patient towards you to rest on your thighs.
	4. Position patient.	1. Clear patient's lower arm away from body. 2. Place upper arm flexed alongside patient's head. 3. Draw patient's upper leg upwards with the knee flexed at right angles. 4. Tilt patient's head.
	5. Check.	1. Firm posture. 2. Check airway and breathing.

Notes

When choosing the preferred side, consider the patient's injuries. If a lower limb is fractured, it is more appropriate to turn the patient so that the fractured limb is underneath and supported.

CONTROLLING EXTERNAL BLEEDING TO A LIMB

Equipment

Combined pad and bandage
Patient

Stages	Key points
1. Apply direct pressure.	1. Look for foreign objects and remove if possible. 2. Grasp the wound with your hand. 3. Elevate the limb to aid in control of bleeding.
2. Rest the patient.	1. Place in a position of comfort. 2. Maintain elevation of the limb. 3. Reassure and inform.
3. Apply combined pad and bandage.	1. Place pad over the wound with the tail medially and the drum (upwards) to the lateral side. 2. Make a fixing turn with the tail around the limb and diagonally over the pad. 3. Cover the pad with overlapping turns until about 20 cm of bandage remains.
4. Secure the bandage.	1. Tie the ends of the bandage together.
5. Immobilise limb.	1. Anatomical or adjacent limb splinting.
6. Check.	1. Comfort. 2. Firm support. 3. Check distal pulse.

Notes

Always wear gloves to avoid 'blood to blood' contact. If a foreign body is embedded in the wound and cannot be removed without causing further damage, either cut a hole in the pad or use two pads to surround the object.

BACK BLOWS

Equipment	Stages	Key points
Patient Suction	1. Position patient.	**Conscious:** 1. Lean the patient over with the head lower than the chest. **Unconscious:** 1. Kneel alongside the patient. 2. Roll the patient onto side over your thigh. 3. Maintain a head low posture.
	2. Apply back blows.	1. Use the heel of one hand. 2. Give 4 to 6 sharp blows rapidly and forcefully between shoulder blades.
	3. Check.	1. Airway: • the patient may cough up the foreign matter. • use finger sweeps to help clear the mouth. 2. Suction if required to remove fluids. 3. If clear, check breathing. 4. If not clear, apply abdominal thrusts.

Notes

Options to consider to achieve a head low position when leaning the patient over are:
• over the back of a chair
• over the edge of a table or bed.

If the victim is a young child, lean the child over your arm, head low.

ABDOMINAL THRUSTS

Equipment	Stages	Key points
Manikin	1. Position self and patient.	1. Stand behind the patient. 2. Wrap your arms around patient's trunk. 3. Place one fist, the thumb and index finger against the patient's abdomen; the palm at right angles, just above the umbilicus. 4. Grip fist with other hand. 5. Ensure fist is over epigastrium, *below* xyphisternum.
	2. Apply abdominal thrusts.	1. Press abdomen with quick inward and upward thrusts 4 times rapidly. 2. Time thrusts with exhalations if discernible.
	3. Check for expulsion.	1. Finger sweeps. 2. Look, listen and feel for air movement. 3. If no expulsion, repeat abdominal thrusts.

Notes

If the patient is unconscious, place supine and straddle at the hips, facing the patient. Place the heal of one hand on the abdomen just above the umbilicus and the other hand on top. Apply thrusts as described above. If the second application of thrusts is not successful, consider laryngoscopy.

DANGER

This procedure is not without hazard. Injury to underlying organs and structures have been reported. It is not recommended in pregnancy or extreme obesity.

This procedure is best practised on a manikin as it is potentially dangerous to do so on a non-choking person. If no manikin is available, practise with caution and *use no force* on the person during the training session.

EXPIRED AIR RESUSCITATION (EAR)

Equipment

Manikin

Stages	Key points
1. Check and clear airway.	1. Manual airway clearance.
2. Check breathing.	1. Look, listen, feel.
Breathing is absent. 3. Position patient.	1. Supine position.
4. Position self.	1. Kneel alongside patient's head.
5. Ventilate patient.	1. Head tilt/jaw support. 2. Seal patient's nostrils. 3. Support chin with other hand keeping patient's mouth slightly open. 4. Take a deep breath and seal your mouth over patient's mouth. 5. Exhale to inflate patient's lungs. and remove your mouth. 6. Ventilate 5★ times without pausing for lung deflation.
6. Check pulse.	1. Carotid pulse.
Pulse present, but no breathing. 7. Continue ventilations.	1. 12-15 full breaths per minute. 2. Periodically check if breathing returns.
8. If breathing returns.	1. Assist breathing until spontaneous. 2. Place in a stable side position to maintain airway.

Notes

★ Initial inflations vary. Some resuscitation authorities recommend *2 initial inflations*.

E.A.R. for the newborn is modified:
*   cover both the *mouth and nose*
*   use 'puffs' of air to inflate the lungs
*   ventilate at 30 to 60 breaths per min.

Infant—ventilate at 25 to 40 breaths per min.

Child—ventilate at 15 to 30 breaths per min.

EAR can also be performed by mouth to nose.

DANGER

Do not use EAR in cases of toxic fumes or corrosive substance ingestion.

CARDIOPULMONARY RESUSCITATION (CPR)—SINGLE RESCUER

Equipment

Manikin

Stages	Key points
1. Check and clear airway.	1. Manual airway clearance.
2. Check breathing.	1. Look, listen, feel.
Breathing absent. 3. Ventilate patient.	1. Give 5* breaths.
4. Check pulse.	1. Carotid pulse.
Pulse absent. 5. Position self.	1. Kneel alongside patient's chest.
6. Locate hand position.	1. Use caliper method: • index fingers locate lower end of sternum and supra-sternal notch; • thumbs locate mid-sternum. 2. Place heel of the lower hand on the sternum, thumb to thumb. 3. Ensure hand is not over xyphisternum. 4. Palm and fingers off chest. 5. Place other hand on top of lower hand.
7. Perform chest compression.	1. Keep arms straight. 2. Shoulders over patient's sternum. 3. Apply vertical pressure over sternum—a depth of 4–5 cm. 4. Release pressure to allow recoil of the chest. 5. Maintain constant hand contact with patient's chest. 6. 15 compressions in 10 seconds.

Notes

* Initial inflations vary. Some resuscitation authorities recommend *2 initial inflations*.
The caliper method for locating the correct hand position is one method. An alternative is to run your fingers along the costal margin to locate the xyphisternum. Then place 2 fingers on this process and locate the other hand on the body of the sternum immediately above the 2 fingers. Damage may be done to underlying organs if the hand is incorrectly located or moved during the compression cycle.

8. Ventilate patient.	1. 2 full inflations.

9. Continue CPR	1. Ensure correct hand position.
	2. Ratio of cycle:
	  • 15 compressions
	  • 2 inflations
	3. Minimum of 4 cycles per minute (i.e. 15 seconds per cycle) and maximum of 5 cycles per minute (i.e. 12 seconds per cycle).

10. Check.	1. Assess pulse and breathing every 2 minutes.

CARDIOPULMONARY RESUSCITATION (CPR)—TWO RESCUERS

Equipment	Stages	Key points
Manikin Assistant	1. Position rescuers.	1. Rescuer A at side of patient's head. 2. Rescuer B alongside patient's chest, (opposite rescuer A).
	2. Perform CPR	1. As outlined for single rescuer with rescuer A doing ventilations and rescuer B doing compressions. 2. Ratio of cycle: • 5 compressions • 1 inflation 3. Minimum 12 cycles per minute (i.e. a compression rate of 60 per min.).
	3. Changeover.	1. **Rescuer A:** Complete inflation cycle and move to alongside patient's chest. 2. Locate xyphisternum with index and middle fingers. 3. Wait for 3rd compression and take over 4th and 5th compressions. 4. **Rescuer B:** Complete first 3 compressions and move to patient's head. 5. Ventilate patient at the end of the 5th compression.

4. Continue CPR	1. Ratio of 5:1.
	2. Minimum of 12 cycles and a maximum of 15 cycles per minute.
5. Check.	1. Monitor the pulse during compression.
	2. Check pulse and breathing every 2 minutes.

OXYGEN ADMINISTRATION VIA FACE MASK

Equipment	Stages	Key points
Disposable plastic face mask Oxygen source Patient	1. Prepare patient.	1. Position according to condition. 2. Reassure and explain procedure.
	2. Prepare equipment.	1. Secure mask tubing to oxygen source. 2. Turn on oxygen and set appropriate flow rate. 3. Extend elastic strap. 4. Ensure malleable nose adjustment is opened out.
	3. Apply face mask to patient's face.	1. Hold mask with one hand and stretch elastic strap. 2. Place elastic strap over patient's head and above ears. 3. Gently position mask over patient's face, fitting nose adjustment to seal. 4. Adjust elastic strap to support mask in position, but not too tight.
	4. Secure tubing.	1. Loop tubing and secure to patient's clothing to prevent dislodgement.
	5. Check.	1. Correct oxygen flow rate. 2. Ensure comfort.

Notes

The 'Hudson' type plastic face mask will deliver an oxygen concentration of about 60% at a flow rate of 8 L per minute. Flow rates below 5 L per minute will cause carbon dioxide retention in the mask and therefore re-breathing.

OXYGEN ADMINISTRATION VIA NASAL CANNULA

Equipment

Oxygen cannula
Oxygen source
Patient

Stages	Key points
1. Prepare patient.	1. Position according to condition. 2. Reassure and explain procedure.
2. Prepare equipment.	1. Secure cannula tubing to oxygen source. 2. Turn on oxygen and set appropriate flow rate. 3. Extend elastic strap.
3. Apply cannula to patient's nose.	1. Hold cannula and extend elastic strap. 2. Place elastic strap over patient's head and above ears. 3. Insert nasal prongs into nostrils. 4. Adjust elastic strap to support cannula in position but not too tight.
4. Secure tubing.	1. Loop tubing and secure to patient's clothing to prevent dislodgement.
5. Check.	1. Correct flow rate. 2. Ensure comfort.

Notes

The maximum flow rate is 6 L per minute. Higher flow rates will irritate the nasal mucousa and produce discomfort. Oxygen cannulae will deliver an oxygen concentration of about 44% at a flow rate of 6 L per minute. A 2 L flow rate will give about 28% oxygen.

APPLICATION OF A VENTILATOR FACE MASK

Equipment

Ventilator face mask
Patient or manikin

Stages	Key points
1. Prepare mask.	1. Select appropriate size mask. 2. Remove cuff cap and deflate the cuff against palm of hand. 3. Allow cuff to reinflate and re-cap. 4. Adjust shape of mask to suit patient's face.
2. Position self.	1. Kneel behind head of patient.
3. Prepare patient.	1. Head tilt/jaw support.
4. Position hand for grip.	1. 5th finger at angle of jaw. 2. 4th and 3rd along body of mandible. 3. Index finger and thumb free. 4. Maintain head tilt/ jaw support.
5. Apply mask to patient's face.	1. Place narrow part over bridge of nose. 2. Manipulate to achieve best fit. 3. Hold mask with first hand, index finger along base and thumb over narrow part. 4. Maintain 5th, 4th and 3rd finger grip on lower jaw. 5. Ensure seal.

Notes

Either hand may be used. The optimum position is behind the patient's head, but if application is required from a side position, twist the hand around to achieve the above described grip. An alternative is to use the thumb on the base of the mask and straddle the narrow part with index and middle finger to achieve a seal.

VENTILATING A PATIENT USING A BAG-MASK VENTILATOR

Equipment

Bag-mask ventilator
Manikin

Stages	Key points
1. Prepare patient.	1. Clear airway. 2. Position supine. 3. Insert OP airway.
2. Position self.	1. At the head of the patient.
3. Prepare ventilator.	1. Select and attach the appropriate size mask to ensure a good seal.
4. Apply mask to patient's face.	1. Use ventilator mask technique. 2. Ensure seal between mask and face.
5. Ventilate patient.	1. Squeeze the self-inflating bag gently to avoid gastric inflation. 2. Observe chest/abdomen movements. 3. Adjust the mask as necessary to maintain a seal.
6. Maintain ventilations.	1. Rate of 12 per min. to afford adequate minute volume.

Notes

Oxygen supplement is added by:
* attaching an oxygen source to the adaptor of the bag.
* attaching the reservoir bag to the system if appropriate (earlier ventilator systems did not use a reservoir—the oxygen was linked directly into the bag).

A guide to ventilation is to squeeze the bag according to the size of the patient:
* adult = full hand
* adolescent = 3 fingers and thumb.
* child = 2 fingers and thumb
* newborn = 1 finger and thumb

VENTILATING A PATIENT USING A DEMAND VALVE VENTILATOR

Equipment	Stages	Key points
Demand valve ventilator Manikin	1. Prepare patient.	1. Clear airway. 2. Position supine. 3. Insert OP airway.
	2. Position self.	1. At the head of the patient.
	3. Prepare ventilator.	1. Select appropriate size face mask and attach to demand head. 2. Select correct setting (child/adult). 3. Open oxygen cylinder.
	4. Apply mask to patient's face.	1. Use ventilator mask technique. 2. Ensure seal between mask and face.
	5. Ventilate patient.	1. Depress demand button/lever. 2. Observe chest/abdomen movements. 3. Release demand button/lever to allow exhalation. 4. Adjust seal as necessary.
	6. Maintain ventilation.	1. Repeat ventilations at a rate of 12 per min. to afford adequate minute volume.

Notes

There is a risk of over-inflating using this positive pressure system. Observation of chest/abdominal movements is essential to maintain a normal respiratory cycle.

VENTILATING A PATIENT USING A SOFT BAG VENTILATOR (OXY-RESUSCITATOR)

A

Equipment

Soft bag ventilator
Closed-circuit manikin

Stages	Key points
1. Prepare patient.	1. Clear airway. 2. Position supine. 3. Insert OP airway.
2. Position self.	1. At the head of the patient.
3. Prepare ventilator.	1. Select and attach appropriate size mask. 2. Open oxygen cylinder. 3. Set KDK valve to 0.5 L/min. 4. Depress KDK valve to fill soft bag.
4. Apply mask to patient's face.	1. Use ventilator mask technique. 2. Ensure seal between mask and face.
5. Ventilate patient.	1. Squeeze soft bag by 1 hand compression. 2. Observe chest/abdomen movement. 3. Adjust seal as necessary. 4. Recharge circuit as required by depressing the KDK valve to fill bag.
6. Maintain ventilations.	1. Rate of 12 per min. for adequate minute volume.

Notes

If ventilating in the case of toxic gases, the KDK valve should be set at 8 L/minute. The system must be vented by opening the cross valve during each expiratory phase.

RESPIRATORY STATUS ASSESSMENT

Equipment	Stages	Key points
Patient	1. Prepare patient.	1. Reassure and inform. 2. Position of comfort.
	2. Check general appearance.	1. Look for distress, anxiety, fight for breath, exhaustion.
	3. Check patient's speech.	1. Can the patient speak comfortably?
	4. Check breath sounds.	1. Check for cough. 2. Listen for wheeze.
	5. Check respiratory rate and rhythm.	1. Observe and count breathing. 2. Observe movement and note expiratory movement for prolonged phase.
	6. Check breathing effort.	1. Look for use of accessory muscles, intercostal retractions and tracheal tugging.
	7. Check pulse.	1. Palpate radial pulse. Tachycardia usually accompanies acute respiratory distress.
	8. Check skin.	1. Observe colour of face and lips for cyanosis. If dark skin, check mucosa of mouth or conjunctiva. 2. Check for sweating.
	9. Check conscious level.	1. Glasgow Coma Scale.

Notes

A prolonged expiratory phase is a significant indicator of poor respiratory status. While a tachycardia is usually associated with respiratory distress, a bradycardia is indicative of extremis.

SALBUTAMOL ADMINISTRATION BY NEBULISER AND AEROSOL MASK

A

Equipment	Stages	Key points
Nebuliser Aerosol mask, Salbutamol nebules Oxygen source.	1. Prepare patient.	1. Reassure and inform. 2. Position of comfort.
	2. Assess respiratory status.	1. Use 9 point assessment criteria. 2. Measure peak flow.
	3. Prepare equipment.	1. Attach oxygen tubing to 8 litre flow oxygen source. 2. Attach aerosol mask to tubing. 3. Attach nebuliser aerosol mask. 4. Turn on oxygen.
	4. Administer oxygen to patient.	1. Inform patient. 2. Apply aerosol mask to patient's face. 3. Ensure a snug fit and comfort.
	5. Prepare salbutamol nebules.	1. Check nebules are salbutamol at the correct strength. 2. Check expiry date.
	6. Administer salbutamol.	1. Briefly disconnect nebuliser and poor contents of nebule/nebules into nebuliser bowl. 2. Ensure misting. 3. Re-connect nebuliser to mask and instruct patient to breath with mouth open.
	7. Transport patient.	1. Load patient onto stretcher and transport. 2. Continue nebuliser therapy en route. 3. Re-assess patient's respiratory status after 5 minutes of nebuliser therapy.

Notes

The dose of salbutamol is in accordance with service protocol. Peak flow reading taken according to protocol.

SALBUTAMOL ADMINISTRATION BY NEBULISER AND T PIECE

Equipment

Nebuliser
T piece,
Salbutamol nebules
Oxygen source
Cannula.

Stages	Key points
1. Prepare patient.	1. Reassure and inform. 2. Position of comfort.
2. Assess respiratory status.	1. Use 9 point assessment criteria. 2. Measure peak flow.
3. Administer oxygen.	1. Via nasal cannula at 4-6 L/min.
4. Prepare equipment.	1. Attach oxygen tubing, nebuliser and T piece.
5. Prepare salbutamol nebules.	1. Check nebules are salbutamol at the correct strength. 2. Check expiry date.
6. Administer salbutamol.	1. Add contents of nebule/nebules to nebuliser bowl. 2. Disconnect cannula and attach oxygen source to nebuliser at 8 L/min. flow rate. 3. Ensure misting. 4. Instruct patient to place T piece in mouth and breathe normally.
7. Transport patient.	1. Load patient onto stretcher and transport. 2. Continue nebuliser therapy en route. 3. Re-assess patient's respiratory status after 5 minutes of nebuliser therapy.

Notes

The dose of salbutamol is in accordance with service protocol. The cannula may be left in-situ for further periods of oxygen therapy, unless it is causing the patient discomfort. Peak flow reading according to protocol.

PALPATING A RADIAL PULSE

Equipment	Stages	Key points
Patient	1. Prepare patient.	1. Position sitting or reclining. 2. Reassure and inform. 3. Rest patient's arm across chest.
	2. Locate radial pulse.	1. Ventral aspect of wrist. 2. Lateral to flexor tendon. 3. Feel for artery.
	3. Palpate radial pulse.	1. Feel pulsation by light pressure to the site. 2. Count rate for 15 seconds. 3. Note rhythm and strength.
	4. Record.	1. Multiply the 15 second rate x 4 to calculate the rate per min. and record. 2. Record rhythm (regular/irregular). 3. Record strength (strong/feeble).

Notes

The radial pulse may not be palpable in cases of poor perfusion, necessitating carotid pulse palpation.

PALPATING A CAROTID PULSE

Equipment	Stages	Key points
Patient	1. Prepare patient.	1. Reassure and inform. 2. Position sitting or reclining.
	2. Locate carotid artery.	1. Place 3 fingers over the patient's thyroid cartilage. 2. Slide fingers about 4cm to the side of the patient's neck. 3. Press gently inwards & backwards against the neck muscle. 4. Feel for artery.
	3. Palpate carotid artery.	1. Feel pulsation by light pressure to the site. 2. Count the rate for 15 seconds. 3. Note rhythm and strength.
	4. Record.	1. Multiply 15 second count x 4 to calculate the rate per minute and record. 2. Record rhythm (regular/irregular). 3. Record strength (strong/feeble).

Notes

The carotid pulse is the principal 'diagnostic' pulse site in the emergency environment and will normally be present in poor perfusion, when other peripheral pulses are absent or difficult to palpate.

PALPATING A BRACHIAL PULSE

A

Equipment	Stages	Key points
Patient	1. Prepare patient.	1. Reassure and inform. 2. Position sitting or reclining. 3. Rest patient's arm.
	2. Locate brachial artery.	1. Mid point of upper arm. 2. Medial aspect. 3. Groove between biceps & triceps muscles.
	3. Palpate brachial pulse.	1. Feel pulsation with light pressure at the site. 2. Count the rate for 15 seconds. 3. Note the rhythm and strength.
	4. Record.	1. Multiply 15 second rate x 4 to calculate the rate per minute and record. 2. Record rhythm (regular/irregular). 3. Record strength (strong/feeble).

Notes

The brachial pulse is the site of choice for the newborn and infants. The carotid pulse is often difficult to locate.

PALPATING A FEMORAL PULSE

Equipment	Stages	Key points
Patient	1. Prepare patient.	1. Reassure and inform. 2. Position supine.
	2. Locate femoral artery.	1. Place 3 fingers about 3 cm from the symphysis pubis (groin) along the rim of the pelvis.
	3. Palpate femoral artery.	1. Feel pulsation by gentle pressure over the site. 2. Count the rate for 15 seconds. 3. Note rhythm and strength.
	4. Record.	1. Multiply 15 second rate x 4 to calculate the rate per minute and record. 2. Record rhythm (regular/irregular). 3. Record strength (strong/feeble).

Notes

The femoral pulse site is not frequently used in pre-hospital care, but may be the only major site accessible in the management of the trapped patient.

MEASURING AND RECORDING BLOOD PRESSURE BY PALPATION

A

Equipment	Stages	Key points
Sphygmomanometer Patient	1. Prepare patient.	1. Reassure and inform. 2. Position at rest. 3. Expose upper arm. 4. Ensure the arm is at the level of the heart.
	2. Apply sphygmomanometer.	1. Place cuff on arm 2.5 cm above elbow. 2. Align bladder mark to medial aspect of the arm. 3. Wrap cuff around the arm. 4. Secure cuff firmly into position with velcro or clip.
	3. Locate radial pulse.	1. Refer page 267 2. Maintain feel.
	4. Measure pressure.	1. Close screw valve and inflate cuff with bulb. 2. Note when pulse is lost and inflate a further 20 mmHg. 3. Gradually deflate cuff by opening the screw valve. 4. Note the pressure when the pulse is again felt. 5. Complete deflation of cuff and remove.
	5. Record.	1. To nearest 5 mmHg.

Notes

The measurement of *systolic blood pressure* by palpation is adequate in pre-hospital care. There is no significant benefit gained from auscultation, using a stethoscope. Blood pressure should be recorded indicating the method used, e.g., 120 palp.

ADMINISTRATION OF ENTONOX

Equipment	Stages	Key points
Entonox demand unit Cylinder Patient	1. Prepare patient.	1. Reassure and inform. 2. Obtain verbal consent.
	2. Prepare equipment.	1. Open cylinder.
	3. Administer Entonox.	1. Instruct patient to hold mask over face firmly to seal. 2. Ensure patient's hand does not obstruct exhaust valve. 3. Ensure exhaust valve is clear of other obstructions. 4. Instruct patient to breathe gently and slowly.
	4. Check analgesic effect.	1. Check for response to pain. 2. If patient becomes drowsy or behaves irrationally, cease administration until improved. 3. Record time of use.

Notes

In circumstances where the patient cannot hold the mask (e.g. if the arms are trapped or injured), the rescuer may be permitted in some protocols to hold the mask to the patient's face. However, constant monitoring of the patient's conscious status is necessary. Under no circumstances should the valve be activated manually.

Contraindications
Caisson disease (the 'bends').
Head injury (likelihood of increasing intercranial pressure).

ADMINISTRATION OF METHOXYFLURANE VIA ANALGISER INHALER

A

Equipment	Stages	Key points
Analgiser inhaler 6 ml methoxyflurane Patient	1. Prepare patient.	1. Reassure and inform. 2. Check contraindications. 3. Obtain verbal consent.
	2. Prepare analgiser.	1. Unwind fastener cord. 2. Hold analgiser mouthpiece down. 3. Check expiry date of methoxyflurane. 4. Pour 3 or 6 mls into base of analgiser. 5. Shake analgiser to dispel liquid. 6. Wipe mouthpiece.
	3. Administer methoxyflurane.	1. Pass analgiser to the patient. 2. Secure cord to patient's wrist. 3. Explain odour. 4. Instruct patient to inhale by mouth and exhale by nose. 5. Leave diluter hole open for 8–10 breaths until patient accustomed to odour. 6. Instruct patient to cover diluter hole with a finger for higher concentration.
	4. Monitor use.	1. Encourage patient. 2. When analgesia is achieved, discourage continuous use. 3. Record time of administration, dose and effect.

Notes

Maximum dose is 6 ml.
Verbal and written confirmation of use is required.
S4 drug.

Contraindications
Severe renal disease and eclampsia.

ADMINISTRATION OF METHOXYFLURANE VIA IN-CIRCUIT VAPORISER

Equipment

Oxy-Resuscitator
6 ml methoxyflurane
Patient

Stages	Key points
1. Prepare patient.	1. Reassure and inform. 2. Check contraindications. 3. Obtain verbal consent.
2. Prepare Oxy-Resuscitator.	1. Turn cross valve to closed position.
3. Prepare vaporiser.	1. Unscrew vaporiser bowl and remove. 2. Check expiry date of methoxyflurane. 3. Pour 3 or 6 ml into vaporiser bowl. 4. Refit vaporiser and tighten screw. 5. Turn vaporiser setting to 'off'.
4. Establish oxygen circuit.	1. Turn on oxygen. 2. Set KDK valve to 0.5 L/min. 3. Fill 2 L bag and instruct patient to hold mask to face and breathe normally.
5. Administer Methoxyflurane.	1. Advise odour. 2. Turn vaporiser setting to '1' and allow 3-4 breaths. 3. Advance vaporiser through each setting allowing 3-4 breaths each time until fully on.
6. Monitor use.	1. When analgesia achieved, reduce setting to maintain comfort. 2. Record time of administration, dose and effect.

Notes

Maximum dose is 6 ml.
Verbal and written confirmation of use is required.
S4 drug.

Contraindications
Severe renal disease and eclampsia.

PAIN ASSESSMENT

A

Equipment	Stages	Key points
Patient	1. Check description.	1. Kind of discomfort. 2. Past history of the discomfort. 3. Same, worse or better.
	2. Check onset and duration.	1. When discomfort began. 2. What made the discomfort start. 3. Was onset sudden or gradual. 4. What patient was doing at time of onset. 5. Has discomfort changed.
	3. Check location.	1. Ask patient to point to location. 2. Other locations. 3. Has discomfort remained in same location or moved.
	4. Check other symptoms & signs.	1. 'Indigestion', nausea, vomiting, sweating, SOB, bleeding, coughing.
	5. Check relief.	1. Has patient taken anything to relieve the feeling. 2. Did patient do anything to try to relieve discomfort. 3. Did anything help. 4. Did discomfort return and was it the same or different.

Notes

In the best interests of the patient, keep the assessment as brief as possible. Questions must not compromise patient care or promote anxiety.

PERFUSION STATUS ASSESSMENT

Equipment

Sphygmomanometer
Patient

Stages	Key points
1. Check pulse.	1. >100—tachycardia. 2. <60—bradycardia.
2. Check blood pressure.	1. >160—hypertension. 2. <100—hypotension.
3. Check colour.	1. Pallor, flushed and cyanotic indicate perfusion problem.
4. Check temperature.	1. Cold and moist skin indicates perfusion deficit.
5. Check capillary refill.	1. Nail bed pressure: >2 seconds indicates perfusion deficit.
6. Check respiration.	1. Increased/shallow breathing indicate compensatory processes.
7. Check conscious status.	1. Alteration may be indicative of perfusion deficit when considered with other points of assessment.

Notes

While respiratory and conscious status are not direct components in the perfusion status check, they provide the other dimensions upon which a judgement can be made about the total patient.

LEAD-TWO CARDIAC MONITORING (LIFEPAK-5 MONITOR)

Equipment	Stages	Key points
Lifepak-5 monitor/ defibrillator 3-lead patient cable Electrodes Patient	1. Prepare patient.	1. Inform patient of procedure. 2. Position either supine or sitting.
	2. Attach electrodes to patient.	1. Ensure access to chest. 2. Avoid areas of hair or bony prominence. 3. Place electrodes: • RIGHT chest beneath lateral 3rd of clavicle • LEFT chest beneath lateral 3rd of clavicle • LEFT costal margin, mid clavicular line.
	3. Attach patient cable.	1. Plug cable into monitor socket. 2. Connect to electrodes: • WHITE to upper right • BLACK to upper left • RED to lower left.
	4. Monitor patient and record position.	1. Switch monitor on and select lead II. 2. Instruct patient to remain still. 3. Press record switch and run 10 seconds of strip. 4. Press record switch again to turn off recorder.
	5. Record patient details on strip.	1. Check quality of strip. 2. Write patient's surname & initials, sex, date & time of recording.

Notes

If recorded strip is torn from recorder, each subsequent strip requires patient details. If a continuous strip, record time of each strip.

DEFIBRILLATION (DIRECT CURRENT COUNTER SHOCK—DCCS)

Equipment

Monitor/defibrillator
Gel pads
Arrythmia manikin
Cardiac rhythm generator

Stages	Key points
1. Check safety.	1. Make certain it is safe to proceed: • no metal surfaces • no water.
2. Prepare patient.	1. Expose patient's chest. 2. Place gel pads: • right of sternum beneath clavicle. • mid-axillary line below line of left nipple. 3. If electrodes are attached to chest, ensure no contact with gel pads to prevent misdirected current flow.
3. Monitor patient.	1. Ensure power mode is set to 'paddles'. 2. Place apex and sternum paddle electrodes on the appropriate gel pads. 3. Observe monitor display to confirm rhythm for DCCS.
4. Power defibrillator.	1. Set power selector to correct output. 2. Activate charge button. 3. Check light indicator to confirm defibrillator is charged.
5. Defibrillate patient.	1. Check visually for safety to proceed. 2. Call 'stand clear'. 3. Ensure paddles are firm and level on gel pads. 4. Re-check monitor to confirm rhythm. 5. Depress paddle discharge buttons simultaneously.
6. Check rhythm and output.	1. Observe monitor for rhythm change. 2. Replace paddles in cradle. 3. Palpate carotid pulse for output.

Notes

If protocol requires multiple defibrillations, maintain paddle electrodes in position until salvo is completed. Energy settings vary, but as a guide, the initial defibrillation attempt is usually at 200 Joules. Further attempts may be at a higher energy setting (e.g. 360 Joules). Some monitor/defibrillators record automatically when the defibrillator is activated. Ensure that you record a rhythm strip of the event, from indication to defibrillate to the rhythm outcome. Note the time of the defibrillation on the rhythm strip and attach it to the patient record sheet.

APPLYING THE MEDICAL ANTI-SHOCK TROUSER (MAST) SUIT

Equipment	Stages	Key points
MAST suit Air hoses Foot pump Patient	1. Prepare patient.	1. Reassure and inform. 2. Ensure no objects in patient's pockets. 3. Position supine.
	2. Apply MAST suit.	1. Slide MAST under patient gently to correct position. 2. Fasten garment firmly around each leg. 3. Fasten garment firmly around abdomen.
	3. Attach foot pump.	1. Attach air hoses to valve outlets. 2. Attach air hoses to pump. 3. Ensure all valves are closed.
	4. Inflate MAST suit.	1. Open left leg valve and inflate with foot pump until velcro crackles or valve pops, then close valve. 2. Repeat with right leg valve. 3. Open abdominal chamber valve and inflate fully with foot pump until velcro crackles or valve pops, then close valve. 4. Remove air hoses and foot pump.

Notes

If the patient's ventilations are impaired, slowly deflate the abdominal chamber.

IMPORTANT

Do not deflate MAST suit rapidly.

INTRAVENOUS CANNULATION

Equipment	Stages	Key points
IV cannula Tourniquet Alcohol swabs Adhesive tape Gauze (or 'Opsite' dressing) Manikin	1. Prepare patient.	1. Reassure and inform. 2. Locate preferred site on arm. 3. Place arm in low dependent position to assist venous distension.
	2. Prepare cannulation site.	1. Apply tourniquet above cubital fossa. 2. Ensure radial pulse is present. 3. Wipe site with alcohol swab.
	3. Insert IV cannula.	1. Select suitable cannula size. 2. Align needle above vein at 20° angle, bevel uppermost. 3. Advise patient of needle prick. 4. Insert needle firmly through skin until needle is in vein. 5. Check for blood flow into needle hub. 6. Reduce angle of needle and advance tip 4–5 mm into vein.
	4. Advance cannula into vein.	1. Slide cannula gently along needle into vein up to the hub. 2. Release tourniquet. 3. Compress vein with thumb near tip of cannula. 4. Withdraw needle while holding cannula hub.
	5. Secure cannula.	1. Attach IV line or 3-way tap as required. 2. Cover site with sterile dressing.

WEAR GLOVES TO PREVENT BLOOD-TO-BLOOD CONTACT

ASSEMBLY OF AN INTRAVENOUS INFUSION LINE

A

Equipment	Stages	Key points
IV infusion set IV soft pack solution	1. Prepare soft pack.	1. Check type, quantity and expiry date. 2. Remove outer pouch. 3. Check clarity of solution.
	2. Prepare infusion set.	1. Check correct set. 2. Open pack and discard airway needle (not needed). 3. Locate drip regulator near chamber and turn off.
	3. Insert IV set into soft pack.	1. Remove soft pack seal. 2. Remove protective needle cap without touching needle. 3. Hold insert tube between index finger and thumb. 4. Twist needle slightly during insertion. 5. Invert soft pack.
	4. Charge IV line to exclude air.	1. Squeeze drip chamber gently to half fill. 2. Open regulator slowly to fill line. 3. Close regulator when line reached. 4. Do not allow fluid to enter protective cap.

Notes

Always wash hands thoroughly before handling IV equipment to reduce contamination. Do not remove protective cap of the needle until ready to connect to IV cannula.

CONNECTING AN INTRAVENOUS INFUSION LINE TO IN-SITU CANNULA

Equipment	Stages	Key points
IV infusion line assembled Cannula in-situ Tape	1. Prepare tape.	1. Cut 4 strips. 2. Length about 15 cm.
	2. Connect IV line to cannula hub.	1. Remove protective cap from line. 2. Insert line into cannula hub.
	3. Secure IV line.	1. Place 1 strip of tape over line at hub connection. 2. Loop IV line along patient's arm to prevent dislodging of cannula if traction occurs on the line. 3. Secure line with tape strips.
	4. Set drip rate.	1. Open regulator to achieve required drip rate.
	5. Check.	1. Maintain correct drip rate. 2. Check site for swelling or discomfort. 3. Check line and exclude air bubbles as required.

Notes

Swelling and discomfort at the infusion site indicates that the cannula has perforated the vein. The infusion should be stopped, the cannula removed and direct pressure applied over the swelling. A new cannula should then be inserted at another convenient site. If the cannula is inserted in a vein at a joint, (e.g. the cubital fossa), the arm should be splinted to prevent dislodgement of the cannula.

SURFACE EXAMINATION OF LIMBS

A

Equipment	Stages	Key points
Patient	1. Prepare patient.	1. Reassure and inform.
	2. Expose limb.	1. Remove clothing as much as possible. 2. Carefully remove footwear.
	3. Check appearance of limb.	1. Look for altered alignment. 2. Compare opposite limb. 3. Check colour of skin and look for evidence of injury: • bleeding • laceration • abrasion.
	4. Feel limb.	1. Distal to proximal. 2. Feel around limb as well as up. 3. Note swelling, pain & irregular shape. 4. Check skin temperature of limb. 5. Check sensations.
	5. Check mobility of limb.	1. Support limb. 2. Instruct patient to move limb towards support and note effect.

Notes

Limb checking should always be performed 'skin-to-skin', not over clothing. However, discretion is important when removing clothing. Mobility checking requires care. The limb should always be supported in the plane of requested movement.

TRACTION SPLINTING—DONWAY SPLINT

Equipment	Stages	Key points
Donway splint Patient	1. Prepare patient.	1. Reassure and inform. 2. Administer analgesia. 3. Remove objects from pockets.
	2. Prepare limb.	1. Remove footwear. 2. Expose limb. 3. Align limb and maintain support. 4. Check distal pulse and sensation.
	3. Prepare splint.	1. Apply ischial ring to patient's upper thigh to achieve a loose fit. 2. Place splint alongside limb with ankle straps free. 3. Depress air release valve to ensure no pressure in system. 4. Unlock collets.
	4. Adjust straps.	1. Lay out velcro straps. 2. Position lower leg support strap in line with calf on splint arm without pump. 3. Position knee strap proximal to knee with long end over short end. 4. Position upper leg support strap in line with mid thigh on lateral arm of splint.
	5. Apply splint.	1. Raise footplate. 2. Place splint over limb. 3. Attach splint arms to ischial ring pegs and lock by turning splint arms. 4. Position patient's ankle in padded strap with foot against footplate. 5. Adjust lower velcro to ensure padded support high on ankle.

Notes

Pneumatic pressure traction should be adequate to maintain comfort. Application of traction splints is restricted to shaft of femur and upper 3rd of tibia fractures.

6. Secure foot to splint.	1. Cross top straps over in-step with longer end under. 2. Tighten around footplate and secure with velcro.
7. Apply traction.	1. Apply pressure by pump to achieve desired level of traction. 2. Gauge should show reading in green segment. 3. Tighten ischial ring.
8. Secure leg support straps.	1. Feed leading edge under limb, over opposite splint arm and back under the limb. 2. Secure with button fasteners.
9. Secure knee strap.	1. Feed long end over knee and opposite splint arm. 2. Secure with buckle fastener over knee.
10. Secure traction splint.	1. Raise heel stand. 2. Recheck and adjust traction level as required. 3. Lock collets hand tight and a further quarter turn. 4. Release pressure valve until gauge registers zero.
11. Re-check limb.	1. Check colour, comfort, distal pulse and sensation.

TRACTION SPLINTING—HARE SPLINT

Equipment	Stages	Key points
Hare splint Patient	1. Prepare patient.	1. Reassure and inform. 2. Administer analgesia. 3. Remove objects from pockets.
	2. Prepare limb.	1. Remove footwear. 2. Expose limb. 3. Align and support limb. 4. Check distal pulse and sensation.
	3. Prepare splint.	1. Position splint alongside limb. 2. Unlock collet sleeves and adjust length of splint to about 25 cm beyond patient's foot. 3. Position heel stand about 15 cm from foot and leave flat. 4. Position straps 2 above and 2 below level of knee.
	4. Apply ankle strap.	1. Position under heel with padded side against foot. 2. Ensure bottom edge does not extend beyond edge of heel. 3. Grasp 3 rings and maintain manual traction.
	5. Position splint.	1. Support limb and elevate enough to allow splint to be placed under limb. 2. Position splint with ischial ring just below line of ischium. 3. Fold down heel stand.

Notes

Application of traction splints is restricted to shaft of femur and upper 3rd of tibia fractures. Caution should be taken with the application of mechanical traction to avoid over tensioning of the limb. Comfort is a guide to establishing the correct amount of traction.

6. Apply traction.	1. Tighten collets. 2. Attach ankle straps to S-hook. 3. Turn knurled knob until straps are firm. 4. Secure ischial ring strap.
7. Secure limb.	1. Position leg support straps and secure with velcro fasteners. 2. Ensure straps are not over fracture site.
8. Check.	1. Ensure traction to maintain comfort. 2. Adjust as required by unlocking collets slightly and turning knurled knob. 3. Check comfort, colour, distal pulse and sensation. 4. Observe fracture site for swelling and adjust straps as required for comfort.

APPLICATION OF A PILLOW SPLINT TO A LIMB JOINT

Equipment	Stages	Key points
Pillow Triangular or conforming bandages Patient	1. Prepare patient.	1. Reassure and inform. 2. Administer analgesia. 3. Expose limb. 4. Remove footwear if ankle or foot injury.
	2. Position pillow.	1. Place to ensure adequate support distal and proximal to joint.
	3. Secure pillow	1. Tie triangular or conforming bandages around pillow to conform pillow to limb firmly.
	4. Check.	1. Check comfort, distal pulse and sensation. 2. Adjust as required.

Notes

The pillow splint is a useful alternative to rigid splinting, especially where angulation of a joint occurs, which cannot be straightened.

APPLICATION OF A FULL ARM SPLINT

Equipment	Stages	Key points
Full arm splint Patient	1. Prepare patient	1. Reassure and inform. 2. Administer analgesia. 3. Expose arm.
	2. Prepare air splint	1. Unzip splint.
	3. Apply air splint to arm.	1. Maintain support to injury. 2. Position open splint under full length of arm. 3. Wrap splint gently around arm. 4. Fasten zip. 5. Inflate splint by mouth only. 6. Secure air inlet bung.
	4. Check.	1. Check comfort. 2. Check firm support and adjust pressure as required. 3. Check for leaks.

Notes

Air splints should be applied to maintain the limb in the normal position of function. Do not apply to an angulated limb.

APPLICATION OF A FULL LEG AIR SPLINT

Equipment	Stages	Key points
Full leg air splint Patient	1. Prepare patient.	1. Reassure and inform. 2. Administer analgesia. 3. Expose limb. 4. Remove footwear.
	2. Prepare air splint.	1. Unzip splint.
	3. Apply air splint.	1. Maintain support for injury. 2. Position open splint under leg. 3. Ensure heel to end of splint. 4. Wrap splint gently around leg. 5. Fasten zip. 6. Inflate splint by mouth only. 7. Secure air inlet bung.
	4. Check.	1. Check comfort. 2. Check firm support and adjust pressure as required. 3. Observe colour and sensation of limb.

Notes

Application of the full leg air splint is not appropriate for fractures above the knee or where the leg cannot be straightened.

CHEST AUSCULTATION

Equipment	Stages	Key points
Stethoscope Patient	1. Prepare patient.	1. Reassure and inform (if conscious). 2. Expose chest. 3. Position patient semi-recumbent (or supine).
	2. Auscultate chest.	1. Use diaphragm of stethoscope. 2. Check anterior fields. 3. Check posterior fields. 4. Use systematic approach. 5. Instruct patient to inhale and exhale through mouth. 6. Note air entry and exit sounds. 7. Note other breath sounds.
	3. Record findings.	

Notes

Chest auscultation is also used for evaluating heart sounds. However, this should be limited to evaluating heart rate when peripheral pulses are not palpable and detecting distant or muffled sounds in chest trauma, which may be indicative of pericardial tamponade. Differentiation of heart sounds is not useful in pre-hospital care, because their presence will not alter the management of the patient and may delay the treatment unnecessarily.

LARYNGOSCOPY

Equipment

Airway manikin
Laryngoscope
Suction

Stages	Key points
1. Position self and patient.	1. Behind patient's head. 2. Patient supine.
2. Prepare equipment.	1. Check laryngoscope to ensure the bulb is secure and the light is on. 2. Place laryngoscope alongside the left of patient's head.
3. Prepare patient.	1. Elevate patient's head using a small pillow or folded towel. 2. Align the head and neck in the optimal airway position. 3. Apply moderate extension of the head and support the jaw. 4. Maintain 'sniffing' position.
4. Insert laryngoscope.	1. Right hand supporting and steadying patient's head. 2. Pick up and hold laryngoscope lightly by the handle with left hand, thumb along handle. 3. Gently insert blade aiming toward the midline and down extreme right side of the mouth.
5. Inspect upper airway.	1. Check for foreign matter in the oropharynx, looking right/left. 2. Do not angulate the blade. 3. Use suction as required.
6. Visualise vocal cords.	1. Gradually move the blade in, keeping the tongue on the left at all times. 2. Try to position the tip of the blade in the vallecular groove. 3. Exert gentle lifting pressure along axis of handle without angulation.
7. Check.	1. Airway clear—use suction to clear fluids as required. 2. Vocal cords in view.

Notes

If obstruction is seen at any stage, remove with Magill forceps. This procedure is contraindicated in children with croup or epiglottitis.

DANGERS

Damage to soft tissues and teeth is likely if care is not taken when inserting the blade. Gloves should be worn to minimise the risk of infection through contact with body fluids.

FOREIGN BODY REMOVAL WITH MAGILL FORCEPS

Equipment	Stages	Key points
Airway manikin, with obstruction Laryngoscope and Magill forceps Suction Equipment	1. Inspect upper airway.	1. By laryngoscopy (refer previous skill statement).
	2. Prepare Magill forceps.	1. Pick up forceps in right hand. 2. Grip with thumb and 3rd finger, index finger to steady forceps.
	3. Introduce forceps.	1. Place tip of forceps in the groove of the laryngoscope blade. 2. Rotate forceps to correct alignment, maintaining view. 3. Advance tips of forceps along blade with *tips closed*.
	4. Remove visualised foreign body.	1. Keep the foreign body in view. 2. Move tips of forceps to about 2 cm from the foreign body. 3. Open forcep tips carefully. 4. Manoeuvre tips to surround foreign body. 5. Carefully grip the foreign body and remove gently.
	5. Check.	1. Inspect the upper airway. 2. Ensure vocal cords are visualised and clear. 3. Suction to remove fluids as required.
	6. Assess.	1. Check respiratory status.

Notes

The foreign body must be seen before attempting removal. Magill forceps are not used to probe. Wear gloves to minimise infection.

ENDOTRACHEAL INTUBATION

Equipment

Airway training manikin
ET tube
Laryngoscope
Clamp
10 ml syringe
Tape
Ventilator
Oxygen source.

Notes

Intubation must only be performed with the vocal cords in view, otherwise damage may be caused. If there is difficulty in introducing the ET tube, a malleable stylet may be used to help guide the tube. External pressure over the larynx ('cricoid pressure'), may also be used to assist visualisation of vocal cords. If, during auscultation, there is no air entry in one bronchus, withdraw ET tube slowly, while ventilating, until bilateral lung sounds are equally audible.

Air escape from the mouth indicates inadequate cuff pressure. Inflate the cuff a further 4 or 5 ml with the syringe. If air is heard in the stomach, the ET tube is in the oesophagus, not the trachea. Remove the tube carefully and repeat the procedure after adequate ventilation of the patient.

Stages	Key points
1. Prepare patient.	1. Positioned supine. 2. Ventilate with oxygen supplement.
2. Prepare equipment.	1. Select correct size ET tube. 2. Check ET tube cuff inflates and 15 mm adaptor is secure. 3. Check laryngoscope bulb is secure and operating. 4. Place equipment in convenient position near patient.
3. Position self and patient's head.	1. Self behind patient. 2. Elevate patient's head and apply extension to achieve 'sniffing' position.
4. Insert ET tube.	1. Perform laryngoscopy to visualise vocal cords. 2. Using right hand, introduce ET tube • right side of mouth; • under continual vision; • through vocal cords until 2-3 cm beyond. 3. Carefully remove laryngoscope, while holding ET tube in position with right hand to prevent dislodgement.
5. Inflate ET tube cuff.	1. Connect syringe to cuff line. 2. Inflate cuff until expiratory sounds are occluded. 3. Clamp cuff line to maintain cuff inflation.

6. Check air entry to lung fields.	1. Ventilate and check symmetry of chest movement. 2. Check for air leaks at patient's mouth indicating cuff not sealing airway. 3. Auscultate chest with stethoscope for bilateral air entry in bronchi. 4. Auscultate stomach for air sounds to exclude possible oesophageal intubation.
7. Secure ET tube.	1. Prepare piece of tape about 70 cm in length. 2. Secure tape to ET tube at level of patient's lips and tie around head of patient. 3. Insert OP airway alongside ET tube.
8. Re-check air entry.	1. Auscultate for bilateral lung air entry.
9. Continue ventilation.	1. Maintain IPPV at appropriate rate per minute.

NEEDLE THORACOTOMY

Equipment

23G needle
14G intracath
Alcohol swabs
10 mm syringe
10 ml sterile water
Gloves
Adhesive dressing
Manikin (or cadaver)

Stages	Key points
1. Confirm presence of tension pneumothorax.	1. Attach 23G needle to syringe and draw up 5 ml sterile water. 2. Swab insertion site • 2nd intercostal space; • mid clavicular line; • on affected side. 3. Insert needle fully at 90° to chest wall immediately above margin of 3rd rib. 4. Withdraw plunger and observe air bubbling.
Air present 2. Prepare equipment.	1. Remove intracath from packet and cut end of plastic sleeve to create a 'flutter' valve. 2. Remove catheter and needle guard.
3. Insert intracath.	1. Swab insertion site 2. Insert at 90° angle to chest wall in same site. 3. Observe 'flutter' valve to confirm decompression of tension.
4. Secure intracath.	1. Tape hub securely to chest. 2. Use double loop of tape.

Notes

If there is no evidence of air movement through the intracath and valve after 5 minutes, the needle should be removed and the site dressed. If evidence of tension re-develops, the intracath should be re-inserted.

NEWBORN CARDIOPULMONARY RESUSCITATION

Equipment

Neonate manikin
Bag/mask ventilator
Oxygen source

Stages	Key points
1. Check and clear airway.	1. Manual airway clearance.
2. Check breathing.	1. Look, listen and feel.
Breathing absent 3. Ventilate patient.	1. Give 5 ventilations with bag/mask resuscitator (with oxygen supplement).
4. Check pulse.	1. Brachial pulse.
Pulse absent 5. Position self.	1. Kneel to side of patient.
6. Locate hand position.	1. Mid sternum. 2. Place 2 or 3 fingers.
7. Perform chest compression.	1. Vertical pressure over sternum to a depth of 2 cm. 2. Release pressure to allow return to normal position. 3. Maintain finger contact with chest. 4. Apply 15 chest compressions in 6-8 seconds.
8. Ventilate patient.	1. Give 2 full inflations by bag/mask ventilator.
9. Continue CPR.	1. Ensure correct finger position. 2. Ratio of cycle: 15 compressions 2 ventilations. 3. Rate of cycles per minute should be a minimum of 8 and a maximum of 10.

Notes

The rate of compressions in each cycle should be 100–120 per minute.

APPENDIX B
Answers

CHAPTER 2

Case history

1. Possible blunt trauma to more than one body region and likelihood of long bone fracture(s), especially lower limbs.
2. No immediate hazard with fire brigade and police in attendance. However, personal risk may exist because of blood or body fluids—therefore wear gloves.
3. The patient is not in immediate life threat and vital signs survey can commence.
4. There is strong evidence of hidden injury, probably significant internal bleeding based on poor perfusion and the mechanism of injury, suggesting sufficient force to cause blunt trauma to the internal organs.
5. Yes. The obvious pattern of injury does not correlate to the depressed nature of the physiological data.
6. Potentially significant because of long bone fracture (femur).
7. Yes. The fact that the rider appears to have been thrown from his motorcycle suggests significant injury potential.
8. Yes. They provide evidence to support the depressed physiological picture and an alert to possible continuing bleeding internally.
9. Airway maintenance—left lateral position (with consideration to left leg injury); oropharyngeal airway if tolerated; suction as required. Respiratory support—oxygen therapy via face mask at 8 Lpm. Antomical splinting for legs (using good limb tied to injured limb) and load to the stretcher using a lifting device (lifting frame or scoop stretcher). Head low posture to improve venous return to the heart (autotransfusion). Transport urgently, continuing full physiological observations, noting improvement or deterioration in perfusion and conscious status.
10. History of the incident—car v. motorcycle, patient believed thrown from cycle to road; physiological picture at the scene and whether changes have occurred during transport; physical injuries identified.

CHAPTER 5

Knowledge checks

1. To ensure an air supply line for the body.
2. Filtering, warming and humidifying inspired air.
3. Epiglottis.
4. Thyroid and cricoid cartilages.
5. Second costal cartilage.
6. Bronchi are cartilaginous and bronchioles are smooth muscled tubes.
7. Alveoli.
8. Just beyond the clavicular line superiorly and the diaphragm inferiorly.
9. Penetrating injuries to the shoulder may involve lung injury (pneumo-thorax).
10. Pleural membrane.
11. Cohesion between the layers is important for expansion and recoil of the lungs as the chest and diaphragm move.
12. Inspiration—contraction of the diaphragm and external intercostal muscles increase the diameter of the thorax, creating a decrease in interthoracic pressure, resulting in a pressure gradient between the atmosphere and the alveoli; Expiration—inspiratory muscles relax, decreasing the size of the thorax causing recoil of lung tissue and increasing the interthoracic pressure, resulting in a pressure gradient between alveoli and the atmosphere.
13. Oxygen = about 21%; Carbon dioxide = about 0.04%
14. Each gas in a mixture of gases exerts its own pressure, depending on its concentration.
15. Oxygen = $\frac{21}{100}$ x 760 = 159.6 (160) mmHg

    Carbon dioxide = $\frac{0.04}{100}$ x 760 = 0.304 mmHg
16. That part of the airway in which no gas exchange occurs.
17. Oxygen = $\frac{14}{100}$ x (760 – 47) = 99.8 (100) mmHg

    Carbon dioxide = $\frac{5.5}{100}$ x (760 – 47) = 39.2 (40) mmHg
18. Chemical and nervous factors.
19. Reduction of oxygen at the tissue level below normal physiological norms, despite an adequate perfusion of blood.
20. Reduced respiration and circulatory deficit.
21. Increased respiratory rate—may be rapid and shallow; pallor due to reduced blood supply; cyanosis—a late sign and indicative of extreme hypoxia.
22. Treat the life threatening causes (airway obstruction, significant bleeding); high flow oxygen until evidence of good tissue perfusion returns.
23. Inspiratory phase; expiratory phase; respiratory pause.
24. 12–16 breaths per minute.
25. General appearance; speech; breath sounds; respiratory rate; respiratory rhythm; breathing effort; pulse rate; skin; conscious state.
26. • Combustible materials not permitted to come into contact with cylinders and fittings;
    • No smoking where oxygen cylinders are in use or on standby;
    • Do not subject cylinders to temperatures above 50°C;
    • Valves should be closed when cylinders are not in use;
    • Oxygen cylinders should not be used without a safe and properly fitted regulator valve;

B

- Cylinders should be secured to prevent toppling;
- Never place any part of your body over a valve nor point it in the direction of a person.

27. 6–8 litres per minute.
28. 4 litres per minute.
29. A reversible small airways disease triggered by a wide range of factors, resulting in bronchial hyperreactivity.
30. Bronchospasm; mucosal oedema; mucous plugging.
31. Bronchospasm.
32.
   - General appearance—distressed, anxious, fighting for breath, exhausted;
   - Speech—difficult, often unable to speak;
   - Breath sounds—cough and expiratory wheeze;
   - Respiratory rate—>20 per minute;
   - Respiratory rhythm—prolonged expiratory phase;
   - Breathing effort—marked chest movement, accessory muscles, intercostal retractions and tracheal tugging;
   - Pulse rate—>100 per minute. Less than 60 per minute is a late sign in severe cases;
   - Skin—pale, sweaty and cyanosed;
   - Conscious state—altered.
33. Chronic obstructive airways disease.
34. Loss of elastic recoil of lung tissue, which results in enlargement of the alveoli during expiration, the loss of elasticity causes compression and further collapse of smaller airways, trapping air in the alveoli.
35. Pursed-lip breathing and use of accessory muscles; barrel-shaped chest; cyanosis a feature of severe emphysema.
36. 28% oxygen initially (2 Lpm via nasal cannula). If no increase in respiratory rate after 3 minutes, increase flow rate by 1 Lpm. Further 1 Lpm increments every 3 minutes up to a maximum of 6 Lpm, providing there is no decrease in the respiratory rate. If decrease occurs at any stage, reduce the flow rate by 1 Lpm and maintain until arrival at the emergency department.
37. Fluid shift into the alveoli, which impairs gas exchange; commonly associated with left heart failure following AMI.
38. High flow oxygen and a comfortable sitting posture. If wheezy breathing, salbutamol may help improve air pathways.

Case history

1. Dangers have been eliminated, so the next step is the primary survey to ensure the patient is not in life threat. Check airway, breathing and pulse. A quick check for external bleeding should also be made in the event that the patient suffered trauma at the time of the collapse.
2. High flow oxygen via face mask at 8 Lpm or 100% oxygen via demand ventilator. Maintain in a lateral position and check vital signs.
3. Respiratory signs suggest significant distress with some partial airway obstruction in the smaller airways (bronchospasm) requiring immediate treatment.
4. Potentially time critical and therefore consider transport without delay.
5. Salbutamol via nebuliser and remove wet clothing to reduce hypothermia problems.
6. Continue nebulised salbutamol in-transit until wheeze has ceased. Warm the patient with blankets and use the vehicle heater to maintain a warm environment in the ambulance. Continually assess vital signs for improvement.
7. History of the incident; Vital signs at the scene and initial treatment.

CHAPTER 6

Knowledge checks

1. Mediastinum, an inverted cone-shape with the apex to the left of sternum, resting on the diaphragm at the level of the 5th intercostal space. The base level with the 3rd rib.
2. • Endocardium—smooth inner lining;
   • Myocardium—thick muscular layer;
   • Pericardium—outer layer forming the pericardial sac.
3. Atria—collecting chambers; Ventricles—pumping chambers.
4. The first branches of the aorta immediately above the aortic valve, supplying the heart tissue with oxygen and nutrients.
5. • Atrial systole—0.1 seconds;
   • Ventricular systole—0.3 seconds;
   • Cardiac diastole—0.4 seconds.
6. Arteries and veins. Arteries carry blood away from the heart and veins return blood to the heart.
7. Capillaries.
8. • Tunica intima—smooth inner lining;
   • Tunica media—smooth muscle;
   • Tunica externa—fibrous connective tissue.
9. Veins have a thinner smooth muscle layer and in the extremities, have valves to prevent back-flow of blood.
10. Refer to Fig. 6.4 on page 99.
11. A process of discharge by an electrical impulse in the myocardium, causing the muscle to contract.
12. The reformation of an electrical charge in the myocardium.
13. • SA node—60–80 per minute;
    • AV node—40–60 per minute;
    • Purkinje fibres—15–40 per minute.

Case history

1. Ask the patient to take a deep breath and whether the pain changes as a result. An increase in pain may suggest pleuritic or trauma origin. Ask whether the patient fell or hurt himself just prior to the onset of the pain which might again suggest trauma origin. If there is no evidence of pleuritic or trauma origins, assume chest pain of cardiac origin until proven otherwise.
2. Use the mnemonic DOLOR (refer page 108).
3. Rest and reassure. Posture the patient comfortably, preferably flat to reduce cardiac workload. Administer high flow oxygen and analgesia (after checking for contraindications). Monitor cardiac rhythm.
4. Sinus tachycardia.
5. Ventricular fibrillation.
6. Charge the defibrillator and apply DCCS (according to protocol).
7. 5 compressions to 1 ventilation.
8. Attempt defibrillation again at a higher energy output (i.e. 360 Joules).
9. Provide IPPV with 100% oxygen. Load the patient and transport to hospital without delay continuing IPPV and checking vital signs.

CHAPTER 7

Knowledge checks

1. Soft tissue protection via the meninges; Fluid protection and support via the cerebrospinal fluid.
2. Cerebrum—conscious functions; Diencephalon—sensory interpretation and homeostatic control; Brainstem—primitive functional centres of respiration and circulation. Cerebellum—balance, equilibrium and coordination of movements.
3. Thalamus and hypothalamus.
4. Brainstem and is the centre for motor and sensory controls of circulation and respiration.
5. Continuous with the medulla and extends down the spinal column to the level of the 2nd lumbar vertebra.
6. Posterior columns which provide awareness of the exact position and direction of movement of the body; Lateral spinothalamic columns which convey senses of pain and temperature to the thalamus; Corticospinal column which conveys motor impulses for precise and discreet movements of the body.
7. Eye opening; best verbal response; best motor response.
8. Refer diagram page 151.
9. It is a quantitative and repeatable scale which provides an early picture of the trend in neurological function or emerging dysfunction.
10. • Precise and detailed conscious status assessment;
    • Frequent total physiological status surveys;
    • Details of mechanism of injury;
    • Good airway maintenance and high flow oxygen therapy.
11. Cervical vertebral region—C5 and C6; middle region (thoracic & lumbar)—T12 and L1.
12. • Sensory survey—responses to light touch and pain;
    • Motor survey—movement deficit to extremities.
13. Life threatening problems take priority over spinal injury; move patient in one piece without rotating or twisting; immobilise spine before lifting or moving the patient; lift in the position found and avoid multiple movements.
14. Cerebral thrombus (clot); haemorrhage into brain; cerebral embolus (detached clot).
15. A series of "small strokes" of short duration between which the neurologic clinical picture is normal.
16. Numbness or paralysis of extremities, affecting one side of the body (hemiplegia); headache and confusion, sometimes with inappropriate behaviour (crying or laughing); difficulty in speaking, often slurred speech; altered consciousness; loss of bladder and bowel control; convulsions may occur.
17. Good communication and reassurance—do not assume that the patient cannot understand; protect paralysed limbs; administer oxygen.
18. Hypoglycaemia—low blood sugar; and Hyperglycaemia—high blood sugar.
19. Refer charts page 161.
20. Generalised tonic-clonic seizure or grand mal; Absence seizure or petit mal.
21. Prevent injury during seizure; manage airway by posture during unconscious phase and administer oxygen; transport quietly offering good psychological support.

22. Ingestion, inhalation, percutaneous by absorption, percutaneous by injection.
23. • Ingestion—corrosive: do not induce vomiting; transport without delay. Non-corrosive: induce vomiting; transport expeditiously; if unconscious, do not induce vomiting.
    • Inhalation—remove patient from environment and administer oxygen; protect yourself from contamination; do not use EAR; transport without delay.
    • Percutaneous by absorption—do not use EAR; ventilate with 100% oxygen and transport without delay.
    • Percutaneous by injection—narcotics: oxygen therapy; if in respiratory arrest, ventilate with 100% oxygen; Narcan IV should be administered; avoid accidental needle stick and wear gloves.
    • Percutaneous by injection—venom injection by snake, spider and insect:
        - Snake and funnel web spider—use pressure immobilisation method;
        - Spider—iced water application will reduce pain;
        - Insect stings—to head, neck and mouth—transport in a sitting posture and administer oxygen.

CHAPTER 8

Knowledge checks

1. • Compact bone which appears solid but consists of a microscopic pattern called haversian systems;
   • Cancellous bone has the appearance of a sponge and contains red bone marrow.
2. Long, short, flat and irregular.
3. Synovial—knee; fibrous—sutures of the skull; cartilagenous—symphysis pubis.
4. Body motion, posture maintenance and production of heat.
5. Skeletal muscle, which is voluntary muscle attached to bone to move the skeleton; smooth muscle found in the walls of hollow structures and is involuntary; cardiac muscle, which is the highly specialised involuntary muscle mass of the heart.
6. Direct violence—fracture at the point of contact; Indirect violence—fracture some distance from the point of contact; Muscle contraction—violent muscle action during seizures.
7. Pain, irregularity, deformity, shortening, loss of movement, swelling, discolouration, unnatural movement, crepitus and tenderness.
8. Support proximal end of limb above fracture site; Grip distal end of limb and apply downward traction; If resistance is felt, or patient discomfort increases, stop immediately and immobilise in position found.
9. Anatomical splinting and mechanical splinting.
10. Analgesia before splinting; Splint before moving the patient; Assess distal circulation and sensation before and after splinting; Immobilise joint above and below fracture site; Control bleeding and dress open wounds before splinting; If in doubt, treat as a fracture.

CHAPTER 10

Knowledge checks

1. Painful and regular contractions—cervical dilation to maximum 10cm; Delivery of child; Delivery of placenta and membranes.
2. Reassure mother; Position in lateral or Sims posture; Administer analgesia during contractions as required; Maintain routine observations and perineal inspection; Place midwifery equipment close by; Seek a history; Notify hospital.
3. Once "crowning" has commenced, position mother supine with knees flexed and thighs apart; Prepare equipment and place a towel under buttocks; Place mother in bearing down position on next contraction and instruct to push; Exert downward pressure (flexion) on baby's head; Instruct mother to pant; Break membranes carefully if still intact over baby's head; When baby's face is clear, wipe away blood and mucous from mouth and nose; Aspirate mouth to remove fluids; Check to ensure cord is not around neck; When baby's head turns to one side, place one hand either side with fingers to chin and guide gently downwards to deliver upper shoulder; Guide head upwards to deliver other shoulder; Support neck and deliver body in upward direction; Ensure clear airway and check breathing; Note time of delivery; Clamp and cut umbilical cord.
4. Respiratory rate = 30–40 per minute;
Pulse rate = 120–140 per minute.
5. Appearance; Pulse; Grimace; Activity; Respiratory effort.
6. Displace uterus downward by placing one hand above symphysis pubis; Apply gentle traction downward on the cord; When the placenta is seen, guide cord upwards and use both hands to cradle, twisting it around carefully to complete the delivery of membranes; Place in a container for hospital examination; Massage uterine fundus to ensure firm contraction and prevent bleeding; Clean and dry mother and check for perineal tears; Check uterine fundus every 5 minutes and note vaginal loss—amount and colour.
7. Uterine massage with mother in head low posture and lower limbs elevated; Administer oxygen and transport urgently.
8. Leave alone and transport without delay; If delivery has commenced, support legs and body until delivery is complete; If the head is not delivered in 3 minutes, gently slide index and middle fingers into vagina in a V formation either side of the baby's nose; Push against vaginal wall until head delivers.
9. Place mother in prone knee-chest position and administer oxygen; Place gloved hand on presenting part of baby and push gently to ease compression on the cord; Transport without delay maintaining hand on presenting part to prevent delivery.
10. Fetal development outside of the uterus, commonly in the fallopian tube, resulting in rupture.
11. Newborn (or neonate) = up to 1 month;
Infant = 1 month–2 years;
Child (pre-school) = 2–5 years;
Child = 5–12 years.
12. Body proportions; Airway; Thorax; Respiratory function; Cardiovascular function; Temperature; Immune system.
13. Newborn: RR = 30–40; HR = 120–140; BP = 70.
Infant: RR = 20–35; HR = 80–130; BP = 70.
Child: RR = 15–25; HR = 70–120; BP = 70. (note: BP is lower limit)

14. Be calm, confident and patient; establish eye contact; sit at child's level; use child's name; avoid a lot of equipment and let child play with it first and explain use; talk to child, not just the parent; avoid leading the child; use favourite toy during examination; examine the problem area last.

15. Injuries which are not consistent with the parent's story; injuries inconsistent with the child's motor development; injuries at variant stages of resolution; parent's story is often vague; parent's demeanour is often unusual.

16. Vomiting as in inducing a vomit with an emetic.

17. Induce vomiting and transport to emergency department without delay.

18. Do not induce vomiting, use milk or other fluids to reduce gastric irritation and transport without delay.

19. Characteristic harsh croupy cough with an expiratory stridor (whistling sound).

20. Transport in a sitting position; Do not attempt to examine the throat to avoid antagonism; Oxygen therapy, preferably humidified; Maintain vital signs observation with particular attention to airway and respiratory function; Be alert to the possibility of total airway obstruction.

APPENDIX C
Glossary of terms

This glossary provides a brief explanation of terms used in this text. For a more detailed definition, it is recommended that you consult a medical dictionary.

ABDOMEN The body cavity bordered by the diaphragm above and the pelvis below.

ABDOMINAL Of or pertaining to the abdomen.

ACID A solution with a pH of less than 7.0.

ACIDOSIS An acid-base imbalance in the body: respiratory acidosis—excess of carbon dioxide; metabolic acidosis—excess of lactic acid.

AIDS Acquired Immune Deficiency Syndrome—a severe impairment of viral origin which reduces the body's immune defence system.

ACUTE Severe symptoms of rapid onset and short duration.

AMI Acute Myocardial Infarction—death of the heart muscle due to ischaemia.

ALKALINE A solution with a pH of greater than 7.0.

ALLERGY Sensitivity to a substance which does not affect most people.

ALVEOLI The air sacs at the end of the terminal bronchioles in the lungs. The place in which gas exchange occurs.

ANAEMIA A blood disorder characterised by a reduction in red blood cells or quantity of haemoglobin.

ANALGESIC A pain relieving agent.

ANATOMIC Related to the structure of the body.

ANATOMY The study of the structure of the body.

ANEURYSM Localised dilation of a blood vessel, forming a sac.

ANTERIOR An anatomical descriptive term denoting to the front or a forward part.

AORTA The major artery originating at the left ventricle of the heart.

APGAR The assessment score used for the newborn.

ARTERY Blood vessel which carries blood away from the heart.

ASTHMA A condition producing respiratory distress and consisting of bronchospasm, mucosal oedema and mucous plugging in the respiratory bronchioles.

ASYSTOLE Cessation of cardiac activity evidenced by a straight line ECG.

ATHEROSCLEROSIS The depositing of material inside blood vessels, narrowing the lumen.

ATRIAL DEPOLARISATION The spread of impulses across the atrial myocardium causing contraction.

ATRIOVENTRICULAR NODE A specialised mass of tissue located at the atrioventricular junction of the heart, slowing down conduction of impulses. Abbreviated to AV node.

ATRIUM The upper chamber of the heart. Plural—atria.

AUTONOMIC NERVOUS SYSTEM That part of the nervous system which controls the automatic functions of the body. It consists of two parts: sympathetic or excitor and parasympathetic or inhibitor.

BASE A solution with a pH greater than 7.0.

BIFURCATION Division into two branches.

BLOOD PRESSURE The force exerted by the blood against the walls of the vessels through which it flows. Abbreviated to BP.

BRADYCARDIA A slow heart rate, normally considered to be under 60 beats per minute.

BRAIN The organ controlling body functions and conscious activity. Located in the skull.

BRONCHI The main divisions of the trachea.

BRONCHIOLE The smallest division of the respiratory pathway.

BRONCHOSPASM Constriction of the bronchioles due to muscle spasm.

BUFFER A substance in a solution which minimises the changes in pH.

BUNDLE BRANCHES Part of the electrical conduction system of the heart. The pathways from the bundle of His to the Purkinje fibres.

BUNDLE OF HIS Part of the electrical conduction system of the heart. Located in the septum.

CANNULA A tube used to administer oxygen (nasal cannula) or insert into a blood vessel (intravenous cannula).

CAPILLARY The smallest division of the blood vessels.

CARDIAC Related to the heart.

CARDIAC CYCLE The period of one action phase of the heart—contraction and relaxation.

CARDIAC OUTPUT The volume of blood leaving the heart per minute.

CARDIOVASCULAR Relating to the heart and blood vessels.

CAROTID The artery in the neck supplying blood to the head. Used as the principal diagnostic pulse site.

CARTILAGE The tough material found in joints and forming part of the skeletal framework.

CENTRAL NERVOUS SYSTEM The brain and spinal cord.

CEREBELLUM The part of the brain located below the cerebrum and adjacent to the brain stem. The centre for balance and coordination.

CEREBRAL Of or relating to the brain.

CEREBROSPINAL FLUID The fluid surrounding the brain and spinal cord. Abbreviated to CSF.

CEREBROVASCULAR ACCIDENT A disruption of the blood flow to a part of the brain, due to a haemorrhage, embolism or thrombus in a blood vessel. Abbreviated to CVA and commonly called 'stroke'.

CEREBRUM The largest portion of the brain, controlling conscious and higher functions (thought, memory etc.).

CERVICAL Relating to the neck (cervical spine)

CHRONIC Of long term or duration.

CHRONIC OBSTRUCTIVE AIRWAYS DISEASE A term applied to a group of obstructive problems of the respiratory tract (e.g. emphysema and chronic bronchitis). Abbreviated to COAD.

CONSCIOUS Alert and capable of responding to stimuli within the environment.

CONTRAINDICATED The use of a procedure or drug is prohibited.

CORONARY The name given to the blood vessels supplying the heart.

COSTAL Relating to the ribs.

CROUP A disease of the upper airway in which laryngeal spasm occurs, causing obstruction of the air pathway. More commonly seen in young children.

CRYSTALLOID A protein free solution used in intravenous therapy (e.g. normal saline, dextrose).

CYANOSIS The bluish tinge to the skin caused by low oxygen (hypoxia).

DECUSSATION The cross-over of nerve pathways.

DEFIBRILLATION The use of direct current counter shock (DCCS) to terminate a lethal dysrhythm (ventricular fibrillation).

DEFIBRILLATOR An electrical device capable of delivering direct current shocks to terminate a lethal dysrhythm.

DEPOLARISATION A process of discharge by an electrical impulse in the myocardium, causing the muscle to contract.

DIAPHRAGM The large muscular organ, which separates the thorax and abdomen and forms the major part of the respiratory mechanism.

DIASTOLE The segment of the cardiac cycle in which the ventricles are relaxed and fill with blood.

DISTAL Anatomical term describing position of a part being furthest from a point of origin.

DISTENSION Enlarged or inflated.

DYSPHASIA Difficulty in speaking.

DYSPNOEA Difficult or laboured breathing.

DYSRHYTHM Lacking in or an abnormal rhythm.

ECLAMPSIA A toxic condition of pregnancy.

ECTOPIC Not in the normal position.

ELECTRICAL CONDUCTION SYSTEM The network of specialised masses of tissue which initiates and transmits impulses across the heart.

ELECTROCARDIOGRAPH The graphic display of the electrical activity of the heart. Abbreviated to ECG.

ELECTRODE A contact which senses electrical activity.

EMBOLISM A mobile mass of material in a blood vessel that may result in blockage of the vessel.

EMPHYSEMA Air or gas in tissues. Pulmonary emphysema—loss of the elastic recoil of lung tissue which results in enlargement of the alveoli.

ENDOTRACHEAL Inside the trachea.

EPIGLOTTIS The leaf-shaped projection guarding the airway, preventing the ingress of food or fluids during swallowing.

EPIGLOTTITIS Inflammation of the epiglottis.

EPILEPSY A disease predominantly featuring seizures.

EXACERBATION A worsening of a disease or condition.

EXPIRATORY Of the act of breathing out.

EXTENSION A movement which removes the angles and lengthens a limb or part.

EXTREMITY An arm or leg.

FEBRILE Relating to fever.

FEMORAL Relating to the femur. Femoral artery—the main artery of the thigh and leg.

FEMUR The largest long bone in the body extending from the pelvis to the knee.

FIBRILLATION The quivering, uncoordinated movements of the myocardium.

FLAIL CHEST Damage to the chest wall resulting in multiple rib fracture, each of which is fractured in more than one place.

FLEXION A movement which creates bends and shortens a limb or part.

FRACTURE The loss of continuity of a bone.

GAG REFLEX Spasm of the airway occurring automatically in response to irritation.

HAEMOGLOBIN The pigment in red blood cells.

HAEMOPTYSIS Coughing up blood stained sputum.

HAEMORRHAGE Bleeding.

HAEMOTHORAX Blood in the thoracic cavity.

HEMIPARESIS Weakness to one side of the body.

HEMIPLEGIA Paralysis to one side of the body.

HEPATITIS Inflammation of the liver.

Hg The chemical symbol for mercury.

HOMEOSTASIS A tendency towards stability in the body.

HYPERCAPNIA Excess of carbon dioxide in the blood.

HYPEREXTEND Place in a position of maximum extension.

HYPERGLYCAEMIA An abnormally high blood sugar level.

HYPERPYREXIA A high and sustained body temperature.

HYPERTENSION High blood pressure.

HYPOGLYCAEMIA An abnormally low blood sugar.

HYPOTENSION Low blood pressure.

HYPOVOLAEMIA Low blood volume due to bleeding.

HYPOXAEMIA Low oxygen in the blood.

HYPOXIA Low oxygen at tissue level.

C

IMI An abbreviation for intramuscular injection.

IMMOBILISATION Preventing the movement of a part by securing to an object such as a splint.

INFARCTION Death. A term usually applied to the necrosis of tissue due to loss of blood supply.

INFERIOR A descriptive term used in anatomy to indicate the lower margin of an organ or situated below.

INFLAMMATION The response in tissues to infection or injury.

INFUSION Fluid administration into the circulatory system.

INGESTION Eating or taking in through the mouth.

INHALATION Breathed in.

INSPIRATION That part of the respiratory cycle during which air is taken into the lungs.

INTERCOSTAL Between the ribs. The muscles which are situated between the ribs are called the intercostal muscles. The space between the ribs is referred to as the intercostal space.

INTUBATION The insertion of a tube into the airway as in endotracheal intubation.

IPPV An abbreviation for Intermittent Positive Pressure Ventilation. The use of positive pressure to ventilate a non breathing patient.

ISCHAEMIA Lack of blood to a part.

IVI An abbreviation for intravenous injection. IV is used to abbreviate intravenous and is used in association with infusion to denote fluid placement into a vein.

JOINT The connection of two or more bones. Another word used to describe this is articulation.

JOULE A unit of energy being the work done by a force of one newton acting over a distance of one metre.

KETOACIDOSIS A condition of high blood sugar level in which fat is metabolised to form ketone and acids. Ketones are organic compounds containing carbon and oxygen.

KILOGRAM A metric unit of measurement for weight. Abbreviated to kg.

LABOUR The name of the process of childbirth, in which the muscles of the uterus contract to deliver the child.

LATERAL To the side or away from the midline.

LITRE A metric unit of measurement for volume. Abbreviated to l or L.

LUMBAR The region of the spine between the thorax and pelvis. Also abbreviated to L.

LUMEN The space inside a tube.

MAST An abbreviation for Medical Anti-Shock Trousers.

MEDIAL A term used in anatomy to describe the position of a part which is toward the midline.

MEDIASTINUM The space inside the thorax, between the lungs, in which the heart lies.

MEDULLA The part of the brain stem which contains the motor and sensory centres for respiration, circulation.

MENINGES The soft tissue protective coverings of the brain and spinal cord.

MENOPAUSE The cessation of the menstrual function in women, usually occurring in middle age.

METABOLISM The process by which the body converts nutrients into energy and waste materials.

mg An abbreviation for the metric unit of measurement for weight—milligram.

ml An abbreviation for the metric unit of measurement for volume—millilitre.

mm An abbreviation for the metric unit of measurement for length—millimetre.

MUCOSA A mucous membrane.

MUCUS A secretion that lubricates and protects the surfaces of the hollow tube structures in the body.

MYOCARDIAL Relating to the muscle of the heart.

NAUSEA The sensation which usually proceeds vomiting.

NEBULISER The device used to deliver fluid medication in a fine mist.

NECROSIS Tissue death usually due to loss of blood supply.

NODE A small mass of tissue which may be normal or an abnormal growth.

NORMAL SINUS RHYTHM The normal rhythm of the heart. Abbreviated to NSR.

OCCLUSION Blockage as in coronary occlusion—the blockage of a coronary blood vessel.

OCCLUSIVE Relating to blockage as in air-occlusive dressing for open chest wounds.

OEDEMA Swelling in tissues due to fluid build up in the intercellular spaces.

OROPHARYNGEAL Pertaining to the oropharynx.

OROPHARYNX The posterior part of the mouth between the soft palate and the epiglottis.

ORTHOPNOEA Difficulty in breathing unless sitting upright.

PACEMAKER The site from which electrical impulses in the heart originate. The SA node is the primary pacemaker, being the site from which impulses are emitted at the fastest rate.

PAEDIATRIC Pertaining to children.

PALATE The 'roof' of the mouth—the superior margin of the oral cavity and oropharynx.

PALE Lacking colour.

PALLOR Pertaining to a lack of colour.

PALPATION Assessing a part by feeling with the hand—as in feeling a pulse.

PARADOXICAL The opposite to that which might be expected—as in the chest wall movements of a flail segment.

PARALYSIS The loss of movement.

PERFUSION The blood flow through the tissues of the body.

PERICARDIAL SAC The envelope surrounding the heart, formed by the two layers of pericardium.

PERIPHERAL Relating to the outer surface of the body.

pH The measure of hydrogen particle concentration, which describes the degree of acidity or alkalinity of a solution.

PHARYNX That part of the upper airway consisting of the oropharynx, the nasopharynx and laryngopharynx.

PHYSIOLOGICAL Pertaining to the functions of the body.

PHYSIOLOGY The study of the functions within the body.

PLEURA The two layers enveloping the lungs, covering the outer surfaces of the lobes, the inner surface of the thoracic wall and the surface of the diaphragm.

PNEUMOTHORAX Presence of air in the thoracic cavity.

POSTERIOR A term used in anatomical description to indicate a position behind, or to the back of.

P-R INTERVAL The time delay between atrial depolarisation and ventricular depolarisation as seen on an ECG. Normal time is 0.2 seconds.

PULMONARY Of or relating to the lungs.

PULSE The wave of increased pressure along an artery causing alternate expansion and recoil of the vessel.

PURKINJE FIBRES Part of the electrical conduction system of the heart. The fibres which conduct the impulse from the bundle branches to the ventricular myocardium.

P WAVE The first deflection of the normal ECG which represents atrial depolarisation.

QRS COMPLEX The deflection of the normal ECG which represents the passage of the impulse through the bundle branches to the Purkinje fibres and represents ventricular depolarisation.

RADIAL Relating to the wrist.

RECUMBENT A lying down posture.

REFLEX A response to stimulation by involuntary muscles.

REPOLARISATION The reformation of an electrical charge in the myocardium.

RESPIRATION Gas exchange between the lungs and the atmosphere (external respiration) and at the tissue level (internal respiration).

RESPIRATORY Of or relating to respiration.

RESUSCITATION The act of restoring life systems.

RIBS The bones forming the thoracic wall.

SEDENTARY Inactive.

SEIZURE A convulsion as in epilepsy.

SEPTUM A wall separating a cavity into two parts (e.g., nasal septum and cardiac septum).

SIDS Sudden Infant Death Syndrome.

SIGN Evidence observed during a physical examination.

SINOATRIAL NODE The primary pacemaker of the electrical conduction system of the heart. Located in the right atrium near the junction of the superior vena cava. Abbreviated to SA node.

SINUS BRADYCARDIA A slow sinus rhythm, normally less than 60 per minute.

SINUS TACHYCARDIA A fast sinus rhythm, greater than 100 per minute.

SPHYGMOMANOMETER The device used to measure blood pressure.

SPINAL Of or relating to the spine.

STETHOSCOPE The device used to auscultate sounds.

STRIDOR Harsh, whistling sound associated with upper airway obstruction.

SUPERFICIAL Affecting the surface as in burns.

SUPERIOR A descriptive term used in anatomy to describe a location above.

SUPINE A posture lying flat with the face upwards.

SYMPTOM A feeling described by the patient.

SYNDROME A collection of features which characterise a condition.

SYSTOLE Contraction.

SYSTOLIC Relating to contraction, as in systolic blood pressure—the peak pressure during ventricular contraction.

TACHYCARDIA A rapid heart rate, in excess of 100 beats per minute.

THERMAL Relating to heat.

THORACIC Of or relating to the chest.

THORAX The cavity of the body bordered by the neck and shoulders and the diaphragm, enclosed by the rib cage.

THROMBOSIS Blood clot formation.

THROMBUS A stationary blood clot in a vessel.

TIA Transient Ischaemic Attack.

TRACHEA The main air pathway from the larynx to the bronchi.

TRAUMA Injury.

UNCONSCIOUS A range of states of unresponsiveness.

VALLECULA The groove at the base of the tongue.

VASOCONSTRICTION A reduction in the diameter of blood vessels.

VASODILATION An increase in the diameter of blood vessels.

VEIN A blood vessel returning blood to the heart.

VENOUS Of or relating to the veins.

VENTILATION The act of breathing or the movement of air into and out of the lungs.

VENTRICLE A lower chamber of the heart.

VENTRICULAR Of or relating to the ventricles.

VENTRICULAR FIBRILLATION An uncoordinated tremor of the ventricular myocardium resulting in ineffective contractions and cardiac arrest.

VENTRICULAR TACHYCARDIA A rapid life threatening dysrhythm.

VERTEBRAE The bones of the spinal column.

VERTEBRAL Of or relating to the vertebra.

VISCERAL Relating to an organ as in visceral pleura—the outer covering of the lungs.

VOCAL CORDS A paired structure in the larynx which produces sound.

VOLUNTARY A term used to describe function under conscious control as in voluntary muscle activity.

WHEEZE A high pitched sound characteristic of lower airway obstruction.

Index

I

317

I

I

I

I

070792 W.M.D.